KATHLEEN DODWELL

The Complete Guide to Mast Cell Activation Syndrome

Demystify MCAS: Find your triggers, calm flares, and create a care plan that works

RUST & RIBBON

First published by Rust & Ribbon 2025

First edition

This book was professionally typeset on Reedsy.
Find out more at reedsy.com

Contents

Disclaimer

The content in this book is provided for general educational purposes only. It does not establish a doctor–patient relationship and should not be used as a substitute for personalized medical advice, diagnosis, or treatment. Always consult a qualified healthcare professional before starting, stopping, or changing any medication, supplement, diet, or therapy.

Discussions of medications, supplements, and procedures—including off-label or emerging uses—reflect the author's understanding at the time of publication. Evidence evolves, and recommendations may change. Drug names, dosages, contraindications, and interactions may vary by individual and by country; consult your clinician and local guidelines.

If you have a medical emergency (for example, signs of anaphylaxis such as trouble breathing, swelling of the lips or tongue, or severe dizziness), call your local emergency number immediately.

The author and publisher disclaim any liability for outcomes resulting from the use of information contained in this book.

Acknowledgments

My deepest thanks to Keiryn, who read this manuscript again and again with patience and care—your sharp eye and steady encouragement made these pages clearer and kinder. I'm also grateful to the many doctors and health professionals who have supported me on my own health journey. Your expertise, compassion, and willingness to listen helped me move forward—and gave me the steadiness to write this book. And to Mum, Dad, Michael, and Rick—thank you for giving me reasons to stay, even in the darkest times. Your love kept the lights on.

Introduction

Your body has an incredible capacity to adjust and find balance. It's capable of more than you might think—able to adapt, recover, and let you know when something isn't quite right. Even on days when you feel tired, dizzy, or off-balance, your body possesses a quiet resilience that, with the right care and attention, can help you feel better and return to living a life you love.

If you've picked up this book, you're likely looking for answers, guidance, or a bit of reassurance. Maybe your symptoms seem to appear at random—your stomach one day, skin the next, then stretches of fatigue, dizziness, or heart flutters. Perhaps you've moved from doctor to doctor, gathering test results that don't quite explain what's happening. Or maybe you've finally heard the words mast cell activation syndrome (MCAS) and felt both relief—because there's a name for your experience—and uncertainty about what comes next.

If any of this sounds familiar, take heart—MCAS is still a relatively new conversation in medicine. Many people navigate years of confusion and frustration before diagnosis. Despite these challenges, there is hope and a path forward—one that can bring clarity, stability, and renewed confidence in your life and your system.

MCAS is like fixing a machine without knowing which parts are broken. Mast cells exist throughout the body, so when they misfire, symptoms can appear anywhere—gut, skin, heart, nervous system, or elsewhere. You might look well but feel besieged by symptoms. This disconnect can be isolating, frustrating, and exhausting.

Your experience is real, and how you feel is valid. MCAS does not have to define you. You are more than your condition—you are a whole person with dreams, relationships, and a life worth living. With the right understanding, tools, and support, you can reduce flares, build stability, and reclaim a sense of control over your life.

This book is your companion and guide. You'll find clear explanations of MCAS, treatment options, lifestyle strategies, and actionable tools for creating a plan that works for you. Even small steps like tracking triggers or finding a supportive care team can make a meaningful difference over time.

MCAS is complex, but you are capable, resilient, and deserving of clarity, care, and hope. You have already taken the first step by seeking understanding. With knowledge, support, and practical strategies, it is possible to move forward with confidence, compassion, and purpose. Your journey with MCAS may be challenging, but it can also be intentional, guided, and full of moments that remind you of your strength and resilience.

Why This Book Exists

This book will provide clarity, practical tools, and encouragement for living with MCAS. It will help you understand your system, explore treatment options, and create a personal plan. Return to this guide whenever you need support or want to refine your approach.

Inside, you'll find guidance on:

- Medications that can help steady overactive mast cells.
- Dietary approaches that may ease symptoms and uncover food triggers.
- Natural and complementary therapies that gently support the body's healing.
- Lifestyle changes that reduce daily stressors and improve quality of life.
- Strategies for building a strong circle of support, including healthcare providers, loved ones, and community allies.

Progress is possible. Symptoms can become more manageable. Life can feel steadier. And even with the complexity of MCAS, it's possible to find a rhythm that works for you, supported by knowledge, practical tools, and a sense of being truly understood.

Start today—choose one action or tool in this book and apply it. Remember, your journey is adaptable and uniquely yours. Share your progress, gather support, and shape your healing path with intention.

Understanding the MCAS landscape

Before we dive into specifics, it's important to acknowledge what the path with MCAS often looks like. For many people, it starts with confusion, as symptoms can appear unrelated and unpredictable. You might feel fine one day, only to be knocked flat the next by something as simple as a meal, a change in weather, or a stressful conversation. This unpredictability can make life feel uncertain, even scary.

What often follows is a long and exhausting hunt for clarity. You may go through endless testing, seeing specialists in gastroenterology, dermatology, cardiology, neurology, and more. Each may identify part of the picture, but rarely does anyone connect all the dots. When you finally meet a provider who recognizes MCAS, it's a relief to have an explanation, but a weight in seeing how little consensus still exists around diagnosis and treatment.

The good news is that while the medical community is still learning, many patients have found ways to regain stability and live fulfilling lives. Progress might be gradual, and it often requires trial and error, but it is possible. One of the biggest shifts comes when you begin to see yourself not as a passive recipient of unpredictable symptoms, but as an active participant in your healing journey. That's what this book is designed to help you with.

How to Use This Book

This book is designed to be flexible. You do not need to read it in a straight line from front to back. Feel free to skip ahead to the chapters that address your most pressing concerns, return to earlier sections for a refresher, or revisit the action plan and emotional well-being chapters whenever you need support. Use this book as a resource and companion along your journey.

- **Chapter 1** will help you understand what MCAS actually is, as well as the symptoms and triggers to look for. We'll also talk about the current challenges around diagnosis, so you know what to expect when pursuing medical testing.
- **Chapter 2** will walk through conventional medical treatments: the medications most often used, what they do, and what to consider when starting them. We'll also cover emerging options that some doctors are beginning to explore.
- **Chapter 3** focuses on natural therapies and lifestyle strategies. This includes dietary approaches, supplements, stress-reduction techniques, and environmental changes that can ease the burden on your system.
- **Chapter 4** is about pulling it all together into a personal action plan. Because MCAS is so individual, the most effective plan will always be tailored to you. We'll talk about how to build that plan step by step, how to track your progress, and how to adapt as your needs change.
- **Chapter 5** shares stories about people who've stood where you're standing, found workable paths forward, and built lives that feel safer, fuller, and more their own. Their experiences offer practical ideas, grounded hope, and proof that small changes can add up.

Throughout the book, you'll find a balance of information and encouragement. You'll get the facts you need to make informed decisions, but also the reassurance that you're not alone and that improvement is possible.

The Emotional Side of MCAS

Managing MCAS is more than just medications and diets—it's also about the emotional impact of living with a condition that is often invisible to others. The uncertainty, the trial and error, and the feeling of being misunderstood can take a toll. It's not unusual to feel anxious, frustrated, or even hopeless at times.

Acknowledging this emotional side is important. It's okay to grieve for the way life used to be or feel overwhelmed by the complexity of it all. And it's okay to seek support, not just medical, but emotional as well. Talking with a therapist, connecting with a support group, or simply having a friend who truly listens can make the journey lighter.

You don't need to carry this alone. Part of living well with MCAS is self-compassion and recognizing that your challenges are real. This book will remind you of that along the way.

A Note on Personalization

There's one theme you'll see repeated throughout this book: MCAS is deeply individual. What works for one person may not work for another. Some people find great relief from dietary changes, while others see more progress with medication. Some may need to address environmental triggers, while others focus on nervous system regulation.

This variability means you have options. Instead of following a fixed approach, you can experiment, track, and find the combination that works for you. Build your own toolkit and adjust it as your system and needs evolve.

Finding Steadiness, One Step at a Time

Take a moment. Acknowledge how far you've come, then act—try a strategy, seek support, or set a new target. Steady steps drive real change.

This book won't promise a quick fix—MCAS is too complex for that—but it will give you clear tools, plain-language insights, and encouragement to build an achievable personal plan and make informed choices about care.

Most of all, it will remind you that you're not alone. Thousands are navigating MCAS and finding ways to live full, meaningful lives. With patience, persistence, and the right support, you can too.

So take a deep breath and set aside the overwhelm for a moment. You don't have to solve everything today. Start with small, steady steps toward more clarity, more stability, and renewed hope.

Understanding MCAS – From Symptoms to Diagnosis

Living with Mast Cell Activation Syndrome (MCAS) can feel like navigating a maze. Symptoms may appear in different systems of the body, vary from day to day, and overlap with other health conditions. Because of this, getting to a clear understanding—and an accurate diagnosis—can take time, patience, and persistence. This chapter lays the foundation: what MCAS is, how to recognize the signs, and what the current diagnostic process looks like.

1.1 What is Mast Cell Activation Syndrome?

Mast Cell Activation Syndrome, at its core, is a problem with some of the most important cells in your body: mast cells. To really understand MCAS, it helps to start with the basics—what mast cells are, what they do when they're working properly, and what happens when they go off course.

Mast Cells: The Body's First Responders

Imagine that your system is a city, and your immune system is its security force. Within this system, mast cells act like neighborhood watch patrols—stationed everywhere, constantly on alert, and quick to respond to trouble. They live in tissues throughout the body: in the skin, the lining of the gut, the airways, the blood vessels, and even near nerves.

Their job is to sense when something dangerous or irritating comes along, whether that's a virus, bacteria, allergen, toxin, or injury. When they detect a problem, they spring into action by releasing a burst of chemical messengers. These chemicals include histamine (famous for causing allergy symptoms), prostaglandins, leukotrienes, and many others.

This release is often called "degranulation"—a bit like opening a bag of tiny molecular fireworks. The goal is to create inflammation, which is the body's way of sounding the alarm and rallying defenses. Inflammation increases blood flow, calls other immune cells to the scene, and helps fight off whatever triggered the reaction.

In a healthy system, this response is lifesaving. Without mast cells, you'd be far more vulnerable to infections, toxins, and environmental stressors. They're part of why a mosquito bite swells, why your nose runs when you have a cold, and why your system can quickly fight off pathogens. They're essential guardians.

When Mast Cells Misfire

With Mast Cell Activation Syndrome, the problem isn't that you have too many mast cells. It's that the ones you have don't behave properly. Instead of staying calm until a true threat is present, they become overly sensitive and easily triggered. (1)

You can think of it like a fire alarm that goes off not just when there's smoke, but also when you make toast, take a hot shower, or light a candle. The alarm system is working—it's just working *too well*, to the point of becoming disruptive.

When mast cells release their chemical messengers at the wrong time or in excessive amounts, the result is a cascade of symptoms. Because mast cells are everywhere in the body, those symptoms can show up almost anywhere: the gut, the skin, the brain, the heart, the lungs, or the nervous system.

This is one reason why MCAS can feel so confusing—two people with the same condition may have completely different symptom profiles. One person might struggle mostly with digestive issues, while another experiences flushing, hives, and a rapid heart rate. Someone else might primarily notice brain fog, headaches, and fatigue. All of these can stem from mast cell misfiring.

How MCAS Differs from Mastocytosis

One important distinction to make is between MCAS and another condition called mastocytosis. In mastocytosis, the body produces an abnormally high number of mast cells. These excess cells can often be seen in a tissue sample or bone marrow biopsy, and the condition is typically easier to confirm. (2).

With MCAS, the number of mast cells is usually normal. The issue lies in their *behavior*. They're present in the right numbers, but they're hyper-reactive—firing off chemical messengers too often or inappropriately. This makes MCAS trickier to detect, since traditional lab tests aren't always designed to measure "over-reactivity" rather than cell counts. (3).

Why MCAS is Often Misunderstood

Because MCAS is still relatively new to the medical world, it's surrounded by misconceptions. Many people—sometimes even healthcare providers—dismiss it as nothing more than "bad allergies." While it's true that histamine plays a role, MCAS is much broader than allergies alone. Allergies are triggered by specific allergens, like pollen or peanuts. MCAS reactions, on the other hand, can be caused by a wide range of triggers: foods, medications, environmental exposures, stress, infections, temperature changes, or even seemingly random events.

Another common misunderstanding is that MCAS symptoms must always be dramatic, like life-threatening anaphylaxis. While severe reactions can happen, most people experience subtler, chronic symptoms that disrupt daily life without looking like a medical emergency. This can include fatigue, brain fog, stomach pain, or skin issues that come and go. Because these symptoms overlap with many other conditions, MCAS often goes undiagnosed or misdiagnosed.

There's also the stigma of being told it's "all in your head." When tests come back normal and symptoms are hard to categorize, patients may be dismissed as anxious, overly sensitive, or exaggerating. This can be incredibly discouraging, leaving people feeling unseen and unsupported. Understanding the science of MCAS helps push back against this misconception: mast cells are real, their chemical messengers are real, and when they misfire, the impact is real.

Everyday Examples of Mast Cell Misfires

To make this more concrete, let's look at a few real-life scenarios where mast cells may overreact in unexpected ways:

- **The restaurant dinner:** You sit down and enjoy a nice meal, but within minutes of finishing, your heart races, your skin feels flushed, and your stomach cramps. Nothing about the food was "unsafe" in the usual sense—but something in it triggered your mast cells.
- **The scented environment:** You walk into a store that's heavily fragranced. Almost immediately, you feel pressure in your head, your nose starts running, and you feel lightheaded. For someone without MCAS, the fragrance is just strong. For you, it's a mast cell trigger.
- **The stressful day:** You make it through a challenging day at work, only to crash later with fatigue, hives, or a flare of digestive symptoms. Emotional stress is a well-known mast cell trigger because mast cells communicate closely with the nervous system.
- **The change in weather:** A sudden shift in temperature or a rise in humidity leaves you feeling off balance. Maybe your joints ache, your skin itches, or your breathing feels more difficult. For most people, it's just a muggy day or a cool breeze. For someone with MCAS, that change in the environment can be enough to cause mast cells to overreact.
- **The unexpected medication reaction:** You take a medication that your doctor assures is safe and commonly used. Instead of relief, you break out in hives, feel dizzy, or experience stomach upset. It's not necessarily an allergy in the traditional sense—it's your mast cells responding

unpredictably and releasing their chemical signals in ways that disrupt your system.

These moments highlight how unpredictable MCAS can be. Triggers don't always come from "dangerous" situations. They can come from everyday life—the foods you eat, the air you breathe, the stress you carry, or even the weather outside. And that unpredictability is one of the reasons MCAS can be so difficult to recognize and manage.

The Complexity of Mast Cell Mediators

Mast cells are remarkably powerful because they are capable of releasing many chemical messengers, sometimes all at once. Histamine is the best known, but it's only one piece of a very large puzzle. Other mediators—such as tryptase, prostaglandins, leukotrienes, cytokines, and growth factors—also play major roles in the body's responses. Each of these chemicals interacts with different systems, tissues, and organs, creating a wide array of potential effects. (4).

For example:

- **Histamine** can cause itching, flushing, hives, swelling, or the release of stomach acid, affecting both skin and digestive health.
- **Prostaglandins** may contribute to pain, inflammation, and changes in blood pressure or circulation, influencing everything from headaches to joint discomfort.
- **Leukotrienes** can tighten the airways, which may result in wheezing, coughing, or difficulty breathing, particularly in those with respiratory sensitivities.
- **Cytokines** act as immune system signals and can drive fatigue, brain fog, flu-like feelings, or even mild fever, creating a sense of general malaise that can be hard to pin down.

Beyond these, growth factors and other mediators influence tissue repair, blood vessel function, and immune coordination, further adding to the body's complexity when mast cells misfire. This vast network of chemical messengers helps explain why MCAS symptoms are so varied. Two people with overactive mast cells may have completely different experiences. One person might struggle primarily with digestive issues and rashes, while another experiences fatigue, headaches, and breathing difficulties. Even the timing and combination of mediators released can change from day to day, which is why MCAS often feels unpredictable and frustrating.

Understanding this complexity is key. It highlights why a tailored approach is so important. Recognizing the range of mediators and their effects helps make sense of the wide variety of symptoms people with MCAS experience, and it underscores the need for strategies that address the condition from multiple angles.

The Power of Clarity

Discovering that MCAS is at the root of how you feel can bring a powerful sense of clarity. What once felt like a jumble of unconnected challenges suddenly resolves into a clearer, more coherent picture. There's reassurance in knowing these symptoms aren't random or imagined; they share a common root in mast cell dysfunction, and that knowledge helps make sense of what you've been experiencing.

Understanding MCAS is valuable for more than just explanation—it also gives you the tools to move forward. When you know that MCAS is a real, recognized condition, even if still evolving in the medical world, you gain the confidence to advocate for yourself. You're better equipped to ask the right questions, push back gently but firmly if your concerns are dismissed, and seek out providers who take how you feel seriously.

Knowledge also opens the door to possibility. While living with MCAS can feel daunting at first, many people discover that it becomes less overwhelming once they have language for what's happening and tools to track their progress. Having a framework for understanding symptoms can turn chaos into something more predictable, and predictability itself brings relief. Over time, this clarity often allows space for confidence to grow—for making choices, planning ahead, and reclaiming parts of life that once felt out of reach. Just as importantly, understanding MCAS can help you connect with others who share similar experiences, reminding you that you don't have to face this alone. Life with MCAS may bring challenges, but it can also hold moments of steadiness, resilience, connection, and even unexpected joy.

Key Takeaway

MCAS is not "just allergies," and it's not "all in your head." It's a condition where mast cells—the body's first responders—become overactive and release their chemical messengers at the wrong times. Unlike mastocytosis, it doesn't involve too many mast cells, but rather ones that misfire. This can cause wide-ranging symptoms across multiple body systems and is often misunderstood or dismissed.

By learning the basics of what mast cells do, how they misfire, and why MCAS is different from other conditions, you gain the foundation you need to navigate your journey with clarity and confidence.

1.2 Recognizing the Signs and Symptoms

Mast cells are everywhere—stationed in the skin, lining the digestive tract, along blood vessels, in the lungs, and even in the brain. When these cells misfire, they release chemicals that affect not just their immediate area but the whole body. This is why one person might mainly have gut issues, another might have skin problems, and yet another might deal with brain fog and fatigue. Some people experience all of the above at different times.

The variety of symptoms is part of what makes MCAS so hard to spot. Doctors who are trained to look at the body in separate "departments" may not connect the dots between digestive pain, a racing heart, and itchy skin. But when you zoom out, you see the common thread: overactive mast cells.

Let's break down the most common ways MCAS shows up, system by system.

Digestive System

The digestive tract is one of the most mast-cell-dense areas of the body, which makes it a problem area for people with MCAS.

Common symptoms include:

- Stomach pain or cramping, often after eating
- Bloating or gas
- Diarrhea, constipation, or a mix of both
- Nausea or vomiting
- Heartburn or acid reflux
- Food sensitivities that seem to multiply over time

For some people, these symptoms mimic irritable bowel syndrome (IBS) or food intolerances. In fact, many people are initially told they just have IBS, only to later discover that mast cells are driving much of their digestive distress.

Food can be a major trigger. It doesn't always have to be "bad" food—sometimes even healthy foods like strawberries, avocado, or spinach can spark a reaction because of their histamine content or other properties that irritate sensitive mast cells. The unpredictability can make eating stressful, leaving people anxious about what meals might set them off.

Skin

The skin is another mast-cell hotspot, which is why skin reactions are some of the most recognizable MCAS symptoms.

Common skin manifestations:

- Flushing (a sudden redness and warmth, especially on the face or chest)
- Hives (itchy, raised welts that come and go)
- Itching, with or without a visible rash
- Swelling of lips, eyelids, or hands
- Dermatographism (skin welts easily when scratched lightly)

These symptoms may look like allergies, but in MCAS they can appear without a clear allergen. A warm shower, a sudden change in temperature, or even emotional stress might trigger a flare.

Some people describe feeling like their skin is a "signal board," reacting instantly to internal changes or environmental exposures. While these reactions can be uncomfortable and sometimes embarrassing, they're important clues that mast cells are overactive.

Respiratory System

Mast cells line the airways, which means the lungs and sinuses often get caught in the crossfire.

Respiratory symptoms may include:

- Wheezing or shortness of breath
- Chronic nasal congestion or a runny nose
- Frequent sinus infections
- Coughing spells
- Sensitivity to fragrances, smoke, or other airborne irritants

Sometimes these symptoms resemble asthma or chronic allergies. In fact, some people are diagnosed with "asthma" that never seems to respond well to inhalers, later realizing MCAS is the underlying driver.

Because breathing symptoms can be frightening, they're often one of the most distressing aspects of MCAS. Even mild airway constriction can create anxiety, which then becomes another mast cell trigger. It's a cycle many people know too well.

Cardiovascular System

When mast cells release their signals, the effects aren't limited to a single area. Those signals can spread and influence blood vessels throughout the body, often leading to cardiovascular symptoms.

Common issues include:

- Rapid heart rate (sometimes called tachycardia)
- Low blood pressure or sudden drops in pressure
- Dizziness or lightheadedness, especially when standing
- Palpitations (feeling like your heart is skipping or pounding)

Some of these overlap with a condition called **Postural Orthostatic Tachycardia Syndrome (POTS)**, where the heart rate spikes abnormally when standing up. In fact, MCAS and POTS often occur together, likely because both involve nervous system regulation and blood vessel tone. (1).

These symptoms can be especially disruptive, because they can limit activity and make everyday tasks such as walking across a room or taking a shower exhausting.

Neurological System

Perhaps the most misunderstood MCAS symptoms are the ones that affect the brain and nervous system. Mast cells communicate closely with nerves, and when they release their chemicals, the effects can be surprisingly broad.

Neurological symptoms include:

- Brain fog (trouble concentrating, memory lapses, mental fatigue)
- Pain
- Headaches or migraines
- Tingling or numbness in hands and feet
- Sleep disturbances
- Mood swings, anxiety, or depression

Brain fog is one of the most common challenges. Many describe it as if their thoughts are moving in slow motion, or like they're trying to tune in to a radio station that just won't come in clearly. This isn't laziness or lack of willpower—it's a direct effect of inflammatory chemicals impacting the nervous system.

Because these symptoms overlap with mental health conditions, patients are sometimes misdiagnosed with anxiety disorders or depression alone, without recognition of the physical root. In truth, mast cell chemicals can directly alter neurotransmitter activity, meaning the "mind" symptoms are also "body" symptoms. (2).

Common Triggers

One of the defining features of MCAS is that symptoms frequently flare in response to triggers. The tricky part is that these triggers can be extremely individual—what bothers one person might not affect another at all.

Some of the most common triggers include:

- **Foods:** High-histamine foods (like aged cheese, alcohol, or smoked meats), leftovers, additives, or even fresh produce like tomatoes.
- **Medications:** Painkillers (NSAIDs and opiates), antibiotics, or contrast dyes used in medical imaging.
- **Environmental exposures:** Fragrances, cleaning chemicals, mold, pollen,

or pollution.

- **Temperature changes:** Heat, cold, or sudden weather shifts.
- **Stress:** Emotional or physical stress can directly activate mast cells.
- **Infections:** Viruses, bacterial illnesses, or even vaccinations may trigger flares.

It's important to note that almost no one reacts to *all* of these triggers. Identifying personal patterns is part of the MCAS journey—and it often takes careful observation and tracking to see what sparks a flare.

Overlapping Conditions

MCAS rarely exists in isolation. Many people are also diagnosed with other conditions that share symptoms or may be linked.

- **POTS (Postural Orthostatic Tachycardia Syndrome):** As mentioned, the overlap in heart rate and blood pressure regulation makes this a common companion. (3).
- **ME/CFS (Myalgic Encephalomyelitis / Chronic Fatigue Syndrome):** Fatigue, brain fog, and post-exertional crashes often mirror mast cell flares.
- **Ehlers-Danlos Syndrome (EDS):** This connective tissue disorder is frequently seen alongside MCAS, suggesting possible shared mechanisms. (4).
- **Long Covid:** Many people report MCAS-like symptoms—flushing, fatigue, brain fog, food sensitivities—after viral illness, especially Covid-19. (5).
- **Allergies and histamine intolerance:** While distinct, these can overlap with MCAS, adding to the complexity.

Recognizing these overlaps can help patients and doctors avoid chasing separate explanations for every symptom, allowing them to see these symptoms as part of a bigger interconnected picture.

Living With the Unpredictability

A person might wake up feeling fine, only to have a flare hit after breakfast or while walking through a store. The symptoms can shift daily, or even hour by hour, making planning difficult and sometimes leaving life feeling out of sync with everyone else's pace.

This unpredictability isn't just frustrating for the person experiencing it—it can ripple into relationships too. Family members, partners, or close friends may struggle to understand why plans are often canceled at the last minute, or why energy can vanish without warning. Their confusion can sometimes seem like frustration, even though it usually stems from not knowing how to help. It's important to remember this isn't anyone's fault. MCAS doesn't follow a neat pattern, and both the person living with it and the people who love them are doing their best in uncharted territory.

What can make a difference is having language for what's happening. When you can point to MCAS as the reason behind the unpredictability, it brings validation—not only for yourself, but also for those around you. It shifts the story from blame or misunderstanding to one of shared compassion and patience.

Key Takeaway

MCAS symptoms can affect nearly every system in the body, which makes the condition tricky to recognize. Digestive issues, skin reactions, breathing difficulties, heart symptoms, and brain fog can all be traced back to overactive mast cells. Symptoms frequently flare in response to triggers, and many people also live with overlapping conditions like POTS or ME/CFS.

The wide variety of symptoms doesn't mean you're imagining things. It means your mast cells are misfiring in different parts of the body. Recognizing the patterns—and understanding you're not alone—is the first step toward regaining control and finding the right management strategies.

1.3 Diagnosis and Medical Testing

For many people receiving a diagnosis of Mast Cell Activation Syndrome feels like finding the missing piece of a puzzle that's been unsolved for years. Getting to that point is rarely simple. MCAS is still a relatively new and evolving area of medicine, and it doesn't always fit neatly into the checkboxes of traditional diagnostic testing. Because of that, patients can spend years bouncing between specialists, collecting stacks of lab results, and hearing confusing or dismissive explanations before someone finally connects the dots.

Understanding the process of diagnosis—the tests available, their limitations, and what doctors are looking for—can give you a clearer roadmap. It won't necessarily make the process easy, but it will help you feel more prepared, more confident in conversations with your doctors, and more patient with the frustrations along the way.

Why Diagnosis Is So Difficult

In a perfect world, diagnosis would be straightforward: run a test, get a clear result, move forward. MCAS rarely works that way.

There are several reasons for this:

1. **Symptoms are wide-ranging and unpredictable.** Because mast cells are found throughout the body, their impact doesn't follow a neat or predictable pattern. The wide range of symptoms can make it challenging for doctors—especially those trained to focus on one organ system at a time. This explains why it can take years of consultations, tests, and trial-and-error treatments before MCAS is even considered. Understanding this complexity not only validates those experiences but also highlights the importance of advocating for oneself and seeking providers who are willing to look at the bigger picture.
2. **Tests aren't always reliable.** The chemical messengers released by mast cells, called mediators, don't linger in the body very long. They can break

down quickly, meaning that unless a test is done at just the right time (often during or right after a flare), results may look normal even when the person is very symptomatic. (1).

3. **MCAS awareness is still growing.** While research has advanced over the past decade, many healthcare providers were never trained to look for MCAS in medical school or residency. This lack of awareness means patients are sometimes dismissed, misdiagnosed, or told their symptoms are "just allergies" or "all in their head."

The path to a diagnosis may have detours, but it is far from impossible. Awareness of the potential hurdles can help you approach the process with clarity and resilience.

The General Diagnostic Approach

Most doctors who are familiar with MCAS look for four key elements when considering the diagnosis:

1. **Symptoms consistent with mast cell activation.** This means the patient is experiencing problems in more than one body system, such as skin, gut, cardiovascular, or neurological symptoms. For example: hives plus stomach pain, or flushing plus brain fog.
2. **Symptoms are worsened by identifiable triggers.** Common triggers include foods, environmental exposures, medications, or stress. If symptoms reliably flare in response to triggers, that supports the possibility of MCAS.
3. **Laboratory evidence of mast cell mediator release.** This could include elevated levels of substances like tryptase, histamine, or prostaglandins. The challenge is that these markers aren't always elevated, even when symptoms are present.
4. **Improvement with mast-cell-targeted treatment.** If antihistamines, mast cell stabilizers, or dietary changes lead to noticeable relief, that adds weight to the diagnosis.

Put simply: doctors are looking for a combination of history, patterns, test results, and treatment response—not just a single positive test.

Laboratory Tests

Lab tests can be tricky to interpret. Let's look at the most commonly used ones:

Tryptase

- **What it is:** Tryptase is an enzyme stored in mast cells and released when these cells become activated. It plays a role in breaking down proteins and contributes to inflammation and tissue changes during allergic or immune responses. Because it is relatively specific to mast cells, it has become one of the most recognized markers linked to mast cell activity.
- **How it's measured:** Tryptase is measured through a blood test, ideally taken during or within a few hours of a flare, since levels tend to return to baseline fairly quickly. Doctors often compare "baseline" tryptase levels (measured when the patient is stable) with levels taken during an episode, to see if there's a significant rise. This comparison can be important for identifying mast cell–related activity.
- **Limitations:** While tryptase is a reliable marker in conditions like anaphylaxis, where levels often rise sharply, its usefulness in MCAS is more limited. Many people with MCAS have normal or only slightly elevated tryptase levels, even during severe flares. This makes it easy for the condition to be overlooked if only tryptase is considered. A "normal" tryptase result, therefore, doesn't rule out MCAS—it simply means other mediators, symptoms, and clinical context must be taken into account. (2).

Histamine

- **What it is:** Histamine is one of the most familiar and widely recognized mast cell mediators. It's responsible for many of the classic "allergy-like" symptoms—such as itching, swelling, flushing, hives, and nasal congestion. Beyond these obvious reactions, histamine also influences stomach acid production, blood vessel dilation, and even communication within the brain. Because of its broad role in the body, elevated histamine can cause symptoms in multiple systems, not just the skin or sinuses. (3).
- **How it's measured:** Histamine can be measured in both blood and urine. Blood tests are sometimes used to detect elevated levels during a flare, but urine testing is often preferred because it can reflect histamine breakdown products (metabolites) collected over a longer period, which may provide a more complete picture. In either case, careful timing is important—tests are usually most informative when samples are collected soon after symptoms appear.
- **Limitations:** Measuring histamine is challenging because levels fluctuate quickly and can be influenced by many factors, including diet, medications, or even stress. Proper handling of samples is essential: if blood or urine is not chilled and processed promptly, histamine can degrade, leading to falsely low readings. This means a normal result doesn't necessarily mean histamine isn't involved—it simply underscores the need to interpret results alongside symptoms and other laboratory markers.

Prostaglandin D2 (PGD2)

- **What it is:** Prostaglandin D2 is one of the key chemical messengers released by mast cells. It plays a major role in controlling how blood vessels widen or narrow, which is why it's often linked to flushing, headaches, dizziness, and episodes of low blood pressure. PGD2 can also influence smooth muscle contraction and contribute to inflammation, making it a significant mediator in both short-term reactions and ongoing symptoms in people with MCAS. (4).

- **How it's measured:** PGD2 is usually measured through a urine test, which looks for either the chemical itself or its breakdown products (metabolites). Because PGD2 can spike during flares, collecting a sample soon after symptoms occur can sometimes capture clearer results. For many patients, a 24-hour urine collection is ordered, as this provides a fuller picture of how much PGD2 the body produces over an entire day rather than at a single moment in time.
- **Limitations:** Like histamine, prostaglandins are unstable and can degrade quickly if samples are not collected and stored correctly. Urine samples often need to be kept chilled or frozen to preserve accuracy, and even small errors in handling can affect results. (5). Another limitation is that PGD2 levels can overlap between people with MCAS and those with other conditions affecting inflammation or blood vessels, so test results always need to be interpreted in the context of symptoms and other markers.

Chromogranin A and Other Mediators

- **What they are:** Chromogranin A is a protein that can sometimes rise when mast cells are active, though it's not specific to MCAS. It's more commonly known as a marker for certain neuroendocrine tumors, but in some cases, elevated levels can also reflect mast cell involvement. (6). Beyond Chromogranin A, there are many other mediators—like heparin, platelet-activating factor, and various cytokines—that researchers and clinicians may look at to piece together a fuller picture of mast cell activity. These additional markers help highlight just how complex the signaling from mast cells can be.
- **How they're measured:** Most of these mediators are tested through blood draws or urine samples. Sometimes, they're ordered when the more common markers like tryptase, histamine, or prostaglandins don't provide clear answers. Because mast cells release different mediators at different times, looking at several of these markers together can give a more balanced view of what's happening in the body.

- **Limitations:** The challenge with Chromogranin A and other secondary mediators is that their levels can be influenced by many factors outside of mast cell activity. For example, Chromogranin A can rise in people taking proton pump inhibitors (medications for acid reflux), or in those with kidney disease or other unrelated conditions. Similarly, cytokine levels may be elevated due to infections, autoimmune activity, or general inflammation. This makes interpretation less straightforward. These markers can provide useful clues, but they're rarely diagnostic on their own—they're most helpful when considered alongside clinical history, symptoms, and other lab results.

It's worth noting that many doctors recommend repeating tests multiple times, especially if initial results are normal but symptoms strongly suggest mast cell involvement.

Timing Is Everything

Because mast cell mediators can disappear quickly from the bloodstream or urine, the timing of tests is critical. The best chance of catching elevated levels is during or right after a flare. For example:

- If flushing, hives, or dizziness suddenly hit, it may be worth heading to a lab promptly for a blood draw.
- Keeping a standing lab order (if your doctor agrees) can make this possible, allowing you to get tested quickly when symptoms spike.
- For urine tests, collecting samples during a 24-hour period that includes flares may give a more accurate picture.

Even with careful timing, it's possible for results to come back normal. This doesn't mean the symptoms aren't real—it simply reflects the challenge of measuring substances that fluctuate so rapidly.

Why Symptom History Matters

Because tests are imperfect, a detailed symptom history often carries as much weight as lab results. Doctors may ask questions like:

- When did symptoms start, and how have they changed over time?
- Which parts of your system are affected (skin, gut, heart, brain, etc.)?
- Do you notice specific triggers, like foods, heat, or stress?
- Do symptoms improve with antihistamines or other treatments?

Keeping a symptom diary can be incredibly useful. Tracking when flares happen, what you ate, what exposures you had, and what helped can reveal patterns that aren't obvious day to day. Even if tests come back normal, a clear pattern of multi-system symptoms and trigger-response cycles can strongly suggest MCAS.

When Symptoms Aren't Taken Seriously

One of the hardest parts of the diagnostic journey is not being believed. Too often, patients hear comments like:

- "Your tests are normal, so nothing is wrong."
- "This is probably just stress or anxiety."
- "It's just allergies—take an antihistamine and stop worrying."

Hearing these responses—especially after months or even years of disruptive symptoms—can feel crushing. It not only invalidates the very real challenges being faced but can also delay treatment, leaving patients stuck in limbo and doubting their own experiences.

Dismissal doesn't just happen in medical settings. Friends, family members, or coworkers may also struggle to understand symptoms that are invisible or unpredictable. They might grow frustrated, unintentionally question your reliability, or misinterpret flare-related absences or cancellations. These reactions can create tension and loneliness, even when everyone involved cares deeply.

If this has happened to you, know you're far from alone. Many people with MCAS share similar stories, and the fault does not lie with you. The issue stems from gaps in medical training, general awareness, and the unpredictable nature of the condition—not from how you feel, your credibility, or your persistence in seeking answers. Recognizing this can be the first step toward regaining confidence, advocating for your needs, and building supportive relationships that respect the reality of your experience.

Strategies for Handling Dismissal

Even though being dismissed is painful, there are ways to navigate these situations while protecting your confidence and well-being:

- **Document how you feel:** Keeping a detailed log of your flares, triggers, and responses to treatments can make your experience tangible. Dates, times, and descriptions—even notes about severity—help you communicate clearly with doctors, friends, or family.
- **Bring a support person when possible:** A trusted friend, partner, or family member can attend appointments, provide moral support, and help convey your experiences accurately when you're struggling to explain them.
- **Educate gently:** Sometimes people dismiss symptoms out of ignorance, not malice. Sharing reputable articles, patient guides, or even short explanations of MCAS can help them understand what you're experiencing.
- **Set boundaries:** It's okay to step back from conversations or situations that feel invalidating. Protecting your energy is essential, especially when symptoms are unpredictable.
- **Seek supportive networks:** Online or local support groups, patient advocacy communities, or MCAS-focused forums can provide validation, practical advice, and emotional support. Talking with others who truly understand what you're going through can make a huge difference.

- **Advocate with confidence:** When working with healthcare providers, bring your documentation, ask clear questions, and don't be afraid to request referrals or second opinions. Remember that you know your system best. Being persistent is not pushy—it's necessary.

Handling dismissal is rarely easy, but using these strategies can help you feel more empowered, reduce frustration, and build the understanding and support you deserve—both medically and personally. Over time, these tools can turn the experience from one of isolation into a path toward clarity, connection, and more effective management of MCAS.

Practical Tips for Navigating Diagnosis

While the process isn't easy, there are strategies that can make it more manageable:

1. **Keep detailed records.** Write down symptoms, triggers, and responses to medications or dietary changes. The more specific your notes, the more persuasive they can be.
2. **Educate yourself.** Understanding the basics of MCAS testing and criteria helps you ask informed questions and advocate for appropriate evaluations.
3. **Seek out specialists.** Allergists, immunologists, or doctors who specifically advertise experience with mast cell disorders may be more open to considering MCAS.
4. **Bring support.** Having a trusted friend or family member at appointments can help you feel grounded and ensure your concerns are heard.
5. **Be persistent.** False negatives are common. If results don't match your experience, it's reasonable to ask about retesting or additional evaluations.

Growing Awareness

The good news is that awareness of MCAS is steadily increasing. More healthcare providers are beginning to recognize the subtle patterns of symptoms, understand the complexity of mast cell mediators, and consider MCAS as a potential explanation when other tests come back normal. Research, while still in its early stages, continues to grow, producing studies that improve understanding of triggers, treatments, and long-term outcomes.

Patient communities are also becoming increasingly powerful voices in the conversation. Online forums, advocacy groups, and social media networks allow people with MCAS to share experiences, practical strategies, and research updates, helping to accelerate awareness both among the public and within the medical community.

While progress may feel slow at times, it is steady and meaningful. Each year brings new insights, more refined testing protocols, and doctors who approach care with greater empathy and understanding. For anyone navigating MCAS, this growing recognition offers hope—not only that symptoms are being taken seriously, but that the resources, support, and research to guide management are expanding every year.

Key Takeaway

Diagnosing MCAS is rarely straightforward. Symptoms vary widely, lab tests are imperfect, and awareness among doctors is still catching up. But diagnosis isn't just about a lab value—it's about the bigger picture: symptoms across multiple systems, patterns of triggers, lab support when possible, and response to treatment.

If you've struggled to find answers, remember this: how you feel is real, you are not alone, and progress is being made. Diagnosis may take persistence, but with the right tools and support, it is possible to move from uncertainty to clarity—and from confusion to a path toward better health.

Conventional Medical Treatments

When facing MCAS, one of the first questions people ask is: *What can actually help me feel better?* While there's no single "cure," there are a variety of medical treatments that can calm overactive mast cells, reduce symptoms, and make daily life more manageable. This chapter covers the main approaches doctors use, what to expect from them, and how to navigate the process of working with healthcare providers.

2.1 Medications Commonly Used

For most people living with Mast Cell Activation Syndrome, medications are one of the most essential building blocks of daily management. While diet changes, lifestyle shifts, and emotional support all matter, medications often provide the immediate relief that makes everything else possible. They can take the edge off flares, reduce the intensity of reactions, and create a steadier baseline from which healing can happen.

It's not unusual for someone with MCAS to feel both relief and hesitation when the subject of medication comes up. Relief, because finally, there is something that might actually help. Hesitation, because so many of us have been told "your tests are normal" or "it's just anxiety," that we may wonder if anyone will really take our symptoms seriously enough to prescribe what we need. On top of that, many people with MCAS are sensitive to medications themselves—sometimes reacting to fillers, dyes, or even the tiniest dose of a drug that's supposed to help.

This is why it's so important to remember: finding the right medication plan is not about fitting into a standard box. It's about building a personal toolbox, step by step. Most people with MCAS end up with a combination of different medications, layered in carefully over time. And while no single pill is usually a magic cure, together, the right combination can mean the difference between constant flares and a life that feels more predictable and manageable.

In this section, we'll walk through the most common categories of medications used for MCAS: antihistamines (H1 and H2 blockers), mast cell stabilizers, and other supportive options like leukotriene inhibitors, corticosteroids, and epinephrine for emergencies. Along the way, we'll look at how they work, what kinds of symptoms they target, what people often notice in real life, and what to keep in mind when working with them.

Antihistamines

Histamine is one of the primary chemicals released by mast cells, and it can cause a surprisingly wide range of symptoms when it gets out of balance. Many people associate histamine only with seasonal allergies—runny noses, watery eyes, sneezing. But in MCAS, histamine can affect the entire body. It can trigger hives, flushing, headaches, stomach upset, diarrhea, rapid heartbeat, dizziness, anxiety, and even difficulty concentrating.

Because histamine is involved in so many of the most disruptive symptoms, antihistamines are often the very first medications tried for MCAS. They don't stop mast cells from releasing histamine, but they do block its effects, which can make a significant difference in day-to-day life.

H1 Blockers

- **How they work:** H1 antihistamines prevent histamine from attaching to H1 receptors, which are located in the skin, airways, blood vessels, and certain areas of the brain. (1). By blocking these receptors, H1 blockers help reduce classic allergy-type symptoms such as itching, hives, flushing, nasal congestion, and sneezing. They can also help calm some of the effects of histamine on the nervous system, which may reduce headaches, dizziness, or mild anxiety related to mast cell activation.

- **Additional notes:** H1 blockers come in both sedating and non-sedating forms. Sedating versions may cause drowsiness, which can be helpful at night but inconvenient during the day. Non-sedating options are often preferred for daily use because they reduce symptoms without causing significant sleepiness. A large number of people with MCAS find that trying different H1 blockers—or combining them under medical guidance—can help identify the most effective approach for their unique symptom profile.

Common examples:

- Loratadine (Claritin)
- Cetirizine (Zyrtec)
- Fexofenadine (Allegra)
- Diphenhydramine (Benadryl)
- Hydroxyzine (Atarax, Vistaril)

What people notice in real life:

- Relief from itching, hives, and flushing.
- Calming of rashes or skin that feels "hot" or irritated.
- Less sneezing and congestion, especially in environments with lots of allergens.
- In some cases, fewer migraines or less brain fog.
- Sedating types (like diphenhydramine or hydroxyzine) help with falling asleep during restless nights.

Things to consider:

- Non-sedating options (loratadine, cetirizine, fexofenadine) are good for daytime use.
- Older antihistamines (diphenhydramine, hydroxyzine) can cause drowsiness and are sometimes best at bedtime.
- Some people need to rotate antihistamines every few months if one stops working as well.
- Because MCAS patients are sensitive, starting with half a pill or even a few drops of liquid antihistamine can sometimes be more tolerable than jumping into a full dose.

H2 Blockers

- **How they work:** H2 antihistamines block histamine from attaching to H2 receptors, which are most concentrated in the stomach and intestines. (2). By doing so, they help reduce the production of stomach acid and can ease digestive symptoms such as heartburn, nausea, stomach cramps, and discomfort after meals.
- **Additional notes:** While H2 blockers are primarily used to support digestive health, some people with MCAS notice broader benefits, including a reduction in systemic symptoms like flushing or mild skin reactions, since lowering histamine activity in the gut can sometimes influence overall histamine levels in the body. H2 blockers are often used alongside H1 antihistamines to provide a more comprehensive approach to controlling histamine-related symptoms. Different H2 blockers may work better for different individuals, so guidance from a healthcare provider can help identify the most effective choice.

Common examples:

- Famotidine (Pepcid)
- Ranitidine (Zantac – mostly withdrawn from markets)
- Cimetidine (Tagamet)
- Nizatidine (Axid)

What people notice in real life:

- Less heartburn and acid reflux.
- Decreased nausea or stomach pain after eating.
- Fewer episodes of diarrhea or urgency.
- Sometimes improvement in flushing or general "flare" symptoms.

Things to consider:

- Famotidine is generally considered the gentlest and most widely tolerated.
- Nizatidine can be another useful option when famotidine isn't effective or available.
- These drugs are often prescribed alongside H1 blockers for more comprehensive relief.
- Long-term use should be monitored, especially for people with kidney conditions.

Using H1 and H2 Together

Taking both an H1 and an H2 blocker together often offers noticeably stronger relief than using either one on its own. H1 blockers help manage symptoms in the skin, airways, and blood vessels, while H2 blockers focus on reducing digestive discomfort caused by excess histamine. When combined, these medications work on multiple fronts, often helping patients feel more balanced and reducing the frequency and intensity of flares.

Medical professionals often consider the H1 + H2 combination a foundational part of MCAS management. It addresses two key pathways of histamine activity, creating a baseline of symptom control that allows other treatments—whether medications, supplements, or lifestyle strategies—to be more effective. While it doesn't eliminate all symptoms for everyone, many patients find it provides a reliable starting point for regaining stability and improving day-to-day comfort.

Mast Cell Stabilizers

If antihistamines work by blocking the effects of histamine after it's already been released, mast cell stabilizers aim to intervene earlier in the process. They help calm mast cells directly, making them less likely to release histamine and other chemical messengers in response to triggers. By reducing the overall activity of mast cells, stabilizers can help prevent flares before they start, rather than just managing symptoms once they appear. This can mean fewer sudden reactions, more predictable days, and a steadier sense of control over their condition for patients.

Cromolyn Sodium

How it works: Cromolyn helps calm—or "quiet"—mast cells, making them less likely to release histamine, prostaglandins, and other chemical mediators that drive MCAS symptoms. (3). By stabilizing mast cells, cromolyn can help reduce both the frequency and severity of flares, supporting steadier days and lessening unpredictability. Its effects are generally preventive rather than immediate, meaning that consistent use over time is often needed to notice improvements. Many people find that when cromolyn is combined with antihistamines, it creates a stronger foundation for symptom management, helping to address triggers before they fully activate mast cells.

Forms: Usually an oral liquid or capsule, but also available as inhalers and eye drops for specific symptoms.

What people notice in real life:

- Calmer digestion—less cramping, bloating, nausea, or diarrhea.
- A reduction in the number of full-body flares over time.
- Subtle but steady improvements in overall tolerance of food and environment.

Things to consider:

- Cromolyn is slow—it often takes weeks or months before benefits are clear.
- Side effects (like nausea or bloating) are common at first but often pass. Starting low and increasing gradually helps.
- Consistency matters—it usually needs to be taken 4 times daily, before meals and at bedtime.

Ketotifen

How it works: Ketotifen is unique because it combines two actions in one. It acts as a mast cell stabilizer, calming mast cells and reducing the release of histamine and other chemical mediators, while also functioning as an H1 antihistamine to block the effects of already released histamine. (4). This dual action can make it especially useful for people with MCAS, as it addresses both the source of the problem and some of the resulting symptoms, potentially providing broader relief and more consistent symptom control over time.

Forms: Oral capsules or compounded liquid (availability varies by country).

What people notice in real life:

- Fewer allergy-type symptoms like itching, hives, and wheezing.
- Gradual stabilization of overall reactivity.
- Improved sleep because of its mild sedating effect.

Things to consider:

- It may cause drowsiness, especially at first. Taking it at night is often best.
- Like cromolyn, it works best when used consistently over time.
- Access can be tricky in some regions, requiring a compounding pharmacy.

Other Supportive Medications

Beyond antihistamines and mast cell stabilizers, other medications can play important supporting roles.

Leukotriene Inhibitors

- **How they work:** Leukotriene inhibitors target leukotrienes, inflammatory chemicals released by mast cells that can contribute to swelling, airway constriction, and other inflammatory responses. (5).
- **Examples:** Montelukast (Singulair), zafirlukast (Accolate).
- **Benefits:** Relief from wheezing, sinus congestion, asthma-like symptoms, and sometimes skin or gut flares.
- **Considerations:** Usually well tolerated, but there is a risk of neuropsychiatric events, so it may not be suitable for everybody.

Corticosteroids

- **How they work:** Corticosteroids are powerful anti-inflammatory medications that help calm inflammation triggered by overactive mast cells. (6). They can reduce swelling, redness, and tissue irritation, and may provide relief for severe or persistent flares that don't respond to antihistamines or mast cell stabilizers alone.
- **Benefits:** Rapid relief during severe flares or before surgeries.
- **Considerations:** Not a long-term solution due to risks (weight gain, bone loss, immune suppression). Best reserved for short bursts.

Epinephrine (Emergency Uses)

- **How it works:** Epinephrine is a fast-acting medication used in severe allergic reactions or anaphylaxis, which can occasionally occur in people with MCAS. (7). It works by rapidly opening airways, tightening blood vessels, and improving blood pressure, helping to stabilize the body during life-threatening flares.
- **Additional notes:** While most MCAS reactions are not life-threatening, some individuals may experience sudden, severe symptoms that require immediate intervention. Carrying an epinephrine auto-injector can provide critical protection and peace of mind. Other emergency medications, such as injectable antihistamines or corticosteroids, may also be prescribed for rapid response in severe flares. Being prepared doesn't mean living in constant fear—it's about having the tools in place so that if a serious reaction occurs, it can be managed quickly and effectively.
- **Practical considerations:** It's important to understand when and how to use these emergency medications, and to have a clear action plan that includes contacting healthcare providers or emergency services as needed. Training in proper use and discussing your personal risk factors with your doctor can help you feel more confident and secure in daily life.

Building a Personal Medication Toolbox

Because no two people with MCAS are alike, most patients end up with a customized plan, often built slowly over months or years. It might look like:

- Morning: cetirizine + famotidine.
- Before meals: cromolyn sodium.
- Emergency: epinephrine auto-injector.

For someone else, it could be completely different. The point isn't to copy someone else's regimen—it's to find what helps you personally stabilize.

Practical Tips for Working with Medications

1. **Start low, go slow.** Especially important for sensitive patients.
2. **Use logs and journals.** Patterns are easier to see when you write them down.
3. **Expect some trial and error.** Not every drug will help, but that doesn't mean nothing will.
4. **Stay consistent.** Stabilizers especially need time to work.
5. **Work closely with your doctor.** Don't be afraid to ask for adjustments or explain what you're noticing.

Real-Life Challenges

- **Access and insurance:** Some meds (like cromolyn or ketotifen) can be expensive or hard to obtain.
- **Doctor education:** Not every provider is familiar with MCAS, so self-advocacy is key.
- **Sensitivity to fillers:** Dyes, preservatives, or even capsules can trigger reactions. Compounding pharmacies can sometimes help.
- **Emotional frustration:** It's normal to feel discouraged when medications don't work right away. Remember—this is a process.

Key Takeaway

Medications for MCAS aren't about "fixing" you—they're about creating a foundation of stability. They give your system a break from the chaos of constant flares so you can live more fully and explore other supportive strategies like diet and lifestyle.

Finding the right combination takes patience and partnership with your healthcare team, but countless people have discovered that once they dial in their medication toolbox, life becomes not only manageable but far more hopeful.

2.2 Other Medical & Emerging Approaches

When it comes to managing MCAS, the most common starting points are antihistamines and mast cell stabilizers. These are often helpful, but they don't always address the full range of symptoms. Some individuals continue to struggle with persistent flares despite using standard medications, while others may notice improvement but still feel the need to explore additional options that could bring further stability or relief. This is where emerging approaches enter the picture.

These therapies are sometimes newer, less conventional, or still under active research. They aren't always easy to access, and their effectiveness can vary from person to person. While some people find them highly beneficial, it's important to remember that these options may also carry more unknowns or potential risks simply because they haven't been studied as extensively. For this reason, it's wise to seek out a healthcare provider who is open to guiding you through these choices—someone who can help balance potential benefits with safety and tailor recommendations to your unique situation.

We'll cover three main categories: Low Dose Naltrexone (LDN), peptide therapies, and other advanced or experimental treatments like biologics and IV therapies. Think of this section as a window into options that are a little less mainstream but increasingly discussed among MCAS patients and progressive clinicians.

Low Dose Naltrexone (LDN)

What it is

Naltrexone is a medication originally developed in the 1980s to treat opioid and alcohol dependence. At full doses (50 mg and above), it blocks opioid receptors in the brain, helping people avoid relapse. But in the late 1980s and 1990s, doctors began noticing something surprising: at very low doses (often between 0.5 and 4.5 mg per day), naltrexone seemed to have immune-balancing effects. This practice became known as Low Dose Naltrexone (LDN).

LDN doesn't work like an antihistamine or a mast cell stabilizer. Instead, it appears to "reset" parts of the immune system, calming down chronic inflammation and improving the way immune cells talk to one another. For conditions where the immune system is overactive, like MCAS, this can be particularly helpful.

How it may help in MCAS

People with MCAS often have a baseline of immune system overactivity. Their mast cells misfire, sending out chemical messengers when they shouldn't. LDN is thought to help by gently modulating the immune system so it doesn't overreact as easily. While we still don't fully understand how it works, researchers believe LDN temporarily blocks opioid receptors, causing the body to increase the production of endorphins and other natural messengers that calm inflammation.

For MCAS patients, this might mean:

- Fewer severe flares.
- Reduced background inflammation.
- More resilience to triggers.
- Better sleep, mood, and energy (as endorphin levels rise).

Evidence and research

Formal research on LDN for MCAS specifically is limited, but studies in related conditions like ME/CFS, fibromyalgia, multiple sclerosis, Crohn's disease, and complex chronic pain have shown positive results. Many of these same symptoms overlap with what MCAS patients experience.

LDN has also gained traction in patient communities. Online forums and support groups are filled with people sharing their experiences, ranging from dramatic improvements to more modest benefits. While not everyone responds, enough people report success that many integrative doctors consider LDN worth trying in MCAS management.

Peptide Therapies

What they are

Peptides are small chains of amino acids—the building blocks of proteins—that act as messengers in the body. They regulate everything from hormone release to immune function to tissue repair. In recent years, doctors have been experimenting with peptide therapies for chronic illnesses, autoimmune disorders, and conditions involving immune dysregulation, including MCAS.

Two peptides in particular have gained attention: BPC-157 and Thymosin Alpha-1.

BPC-157 (Body Protection Compound-157) is a synthetic peptide derived from a protein naturally present in the stomach. Early research, mostly in animal studies, suggests it may play a role in supporting gut healing, promoting tissue repair, and reducing inflammation throughout the body. Because the digestive system is often a major site of difficulty for people with MCAS—whether it's diarrhea, reflux, abdominal pain, or increased intestinal permeability (sometimes referred to as "leaky gut")—BPC-157 has attracted attention as a potential tool for strengthening the intestinal lining and calming inflammatory responses. Some clinicians and patients are hopeful that it may offer benefits not only for gut-related issues but also for broader tissue repair and recovery. However, while the preliminary findings are intriguing, human research remains very limited, and more studies are needed to specifically confirm its safety and effectiveness in MCAS.

Thymosin Alpha-1 is a naturally occurring peptide that helps regulate the immune system. It's been used internationally for decades to support people with viral infections, immune deficiencies, and even certain cancers. (1). In MCAS, Thymosin Alpha-1 may help rebalance immune responses, reducing inappropriate mast cell activation while strengthening the body's ability to handle infections and stress.

Other peptides sometimes considered

- **VIP (Vasoactive Intestinal Peptide):** This naturally occurring peptide helps regulate both gut and lung function. (2). In the digestive system, it supports healthy motility and nutrient absorption, while in the lungs, it relaxes airways and aids oxygen exchange. For people with MCAS, VIP is sometimes considered as a therapy to reduce inflammation and ease both digestive and breathing symptoms.
- **LL-37:** This peptide is part of the body's natural defense system and has strong antimicrobial properties. It helps fight off bacteria, viruses, and fungi, while also playing a role in regulating inflammation. For people with MCAS, LL-37 is sometimes considered as a therapy to support immune balance and reduce the risk of frequent or lingering infections.
- **KPV:** This small peptide has notable anti-inflammatory effects, especially in the skin and gut. (3). It can help calm redness, irritation, and inflammatory reactions in the digestive tract or on the skin's surface. For people with MCAS, KPV is sometimes explored as a therapy to ease rashes, gut pain, or other flare-related inflammation.

Other Advanced or Experimental Treatments

Biologics (e.g., Omalizumab)

Biologics are medications derived from living cells that are designed to target specific pathways in the immune system with precision. (4). One of the biologics most frequently discussed in the context of MCAS is omalizumab (Xolair). Originally approved to treat allergic asthma and chronic hives, omalizumab works by binding to IgE, an antibody that plays a key role in allergic reactions, preventing it from triggering mast cells. By reducing IgE activity, omalizumab can help calm overactive mast cells and decrease the frequency and severity of certain allergic and inflammatory symptoms. For some patients with MCAS, this therapy has provided meaningful relief when standard medications were insufficient, though responses vary, and ongoing monitoring with a knowledgeable healthcare provider is essential.

IV Therapies

- **IVIG (Intravenous Immunoglobulin):** IVIG is a therapy made from pooled antibodies collected from healthy donors. (5). In some people with MCAS, it appears to help stabilize the immune system, potentially reducing the frequency or severity of flares and supporting overall immune balance. Responses can vary widely, however, and research on IVIG specifically for MCAS is still limited. Because it is a more intensive therapy, it is typically reserved for patients with severe or refractory symptoms and should always be administered under close supervision by a healthcare provider familiar with MCAS.
- **IV Vitamin C:** Intravenous vitamin C is sometimes used in MCAS to help calm overactive mast cells and reduce inflammation. (6). Some patients report a range of benefits, including clearer skin, fewer headaches, improved energy, and a greater sense of overall well-being. Because IV delivery allows higher doses than oral supplements, it may have more noticeable effects for certain individuals. Responses can vary, and it's important to work with a healthcare provider to determine appropriate dosing and monitor for any potential side effects.
- **IV Nutrients:** Some people with MCAS benefit from intravenous nutrient therapy, which delivers vitamins, minerals, and other supportive compounds directly into the bloodstream. Custom blends can be tailored to support recovery after flares, replenish deficiencies, and help the body maintain stability. Patients may notice improvements in energy, mental clarity, or overall resilience. As with other IV therapies, responses vary, and it's important to work with a knowledgeable healthcare provider to ensure the blend and dosing are safe and appropriate for individual needs.
- **Ozone Therapy:** Ozone therapy is a treatment in which a small amount of ozone gas is introduced into the body, typically via blood or IV methods. While considered controversial and not widely studied in MCAS, some patients report benefits such as reduced infections, decreased

inflammation, and improved energy. Responses are highly individual, and because research is limited, safety and efficacy remain uncertain. Anyone considering ozone therapy should consult with a healthcare provider experienced in MCAS and closely monitor for potential side effects.

Pulling It Together

Exploring other medical and emerging approaches can feel like stepping into uncharted territory. Some of these therapies, like LDN, are relatively affordable and low risk. Others, like peptides or biologics, can be harder to access and come with higher costs or uncertainties.

The most important things to keep in mind are:

- These therapies are not replacements for antihistamines or stabilizers but add-ons that may help when standard treatments aren't enough.
- Responses vary widely. What works for one person may not work for another.
- Working with a knowledgeable, open-minded healthcare provider is key.
- These therapies potentially carry more or unknown risks.

These therapies represent a source of hope, signaling that the medical community is beginning to explore MCAS with more creativity. They offer potential ways forward for individuals who haven't found sufficient relief through traditional treatments.

2.3 Working with Healthcare Providers

Living with Mast Cell Activation Syndrome (MCAS) often means navigating a maze of appointments, specialists, and confusing medical jargon. One of the biggest challenges isn't just the condition itself—it's finding the right support system to help manage it. Doctors may not always be familiar with MCAS, and the medical system can sometimes feel rushed or dismissive, especially when symptoms don't fit neatly into a box. But remember: you deserve good care, and there are ways to find it. Even if it takes time, persistence, and a little trial and error, it is possible to build a team of providers who understand your needs, respect your experiences, and work with you to create solutions that actually make a difference in daily life.

Think of this section as your roadmap. It will guide you on how to identify doctors, specialists, and other professionals who can support your health; how to communicate effectively so your concerns are taken seriously; and how to develop a long-term plan that fits into the rhythms of your everyday life—not just on paper, but in a way that feels practical, sustainable, and supportive. With the right team in place, managing MCAS can become less overwhelming, leaving space for stability, confidence, and even moments of ease amidst the challenges.

Finding the Right Doctor or Specialist

The first hurdle is often simply finding a provider who knows what the condition is. Many patients describe the early part of their journey as a frustrating cycle: bouncing from one doctor to another, getting half-answers, being told their symptoms are "just anxiety," or being treated for unrelated conditions while the root problem goes undiagnosed. If this sounds familiar, you're not alone.

Where to Start

If you're just beginning, it can help to know which specialties are most likely to be familiar with MCAS:

- **Allergists and Immunologists** – These specialists are often the starting point for MCAS care. While some have extensive experience with mast cell disorders, others may be less familiar. Working with a knowledgeable allergist or immunologist can help ensure accurate testing, proper interpretation of results, and guidance on the most effective treatment options.

- **Hematologists** – More commonly familiar with mastocytosis, but some also have experience with MCAS. They can be helpful in interpreting blood tests, understanding abnormal mast cell activity, and collaborating with other specialists to ensure a comprehensive approach to care.
- **Gastroenterologists** – These specialists can be particularly helpful when digestive symptoms are prominent, such as nausea, diarrhea, or abdominal pain. They can evaluate gut health, rule out other gastrointestinal conditions, and work alongside your MCAS care team to develop strategies that support digestion and reduce flare-ups.
- **Neurologists or Cardiologists** – May become part of your care team when MCAS overlaps with conditions like POTS, migraines, or other nervous system and cardiovascular issues. They can help evaluate symptoms such as dizziness, rapid heart rate, fainting, or nerve-related pain, and coordinate with your other providers to create a comprehensive management plan.
- **Integrative and Functional Medicine Doctors** – While visits with these specialists are not always covered by insurance, they often take the time to explore complex, multi-system issues like MCAS in depth. They may look at diet, lifestyle, environmental exposures, and underlying triggers, and can help coordinate natural and conventional approaches alongside your other healthcare providers.

The reality is that you may not find a single "MCAS expert" in your area. Instead, you may end up with a small team—perhaps an allergist for medications, a gastroenterologist for digestive issues, and a primary care provider to coordinate. That's okay. What matters most is that your doctors are willing to listen, learn, and partner with you.

Red Flags vs. Green Flags

When meeting a new doctor, pay attention not just to their knowledge, but also to how they treat you. A provider who listens carefully, validates your experiences, and communicates clearly can make a huge difference in your care, helping you feel supported rather than dismissed.

Red flags (warning signs):

- Dismissing how you feel as stress or anxiety without further investigation.
- Insisting that MCAS "isn't real" or "too rare to matter."
- Declining to consider treatment options simply because your lab results aren't fully conclusive.

Green flags (good signs):

- They admit what they don't know, but show curiosity and a willingness to learn.
- They ask thoughtful questions about how you feel, triggers, and history.
- They encourage collaboration—between you, them, and other providers.

Communicating Effectively About Symptoms and Responses

Once you've found a doctor who's willing to work with you, the next challenge is making sure they *really hear* what you're experiencing. MCAS symptoms can be overwhelming and wide-ranging. It's easy to forget details in the moment, especially during a short appointment.

The Power of Tracking

One of the most useful tools you can bring to your appointments is a symptom and trigger journal. This doesn't have to be fancy. A notebook, spreadsheet, or even an app can work. The key is consistency.

What to track:

- **Symptoms**: What happened, how severe, how long it lasted.
- **Possible triggers**: Foods, medications, environmental exposures, stress.
- **Timing**: Did symptoms happen immediately, or hours later?

- **Interventions**: Did anything help? (e.g., antihistamine, rest, hydration).

This information gives your doctor a clearer picture and helps them connect the dots.

Speaking Your Doctor's Language

Doctors are trained to think in terms of patterns and evidence. When you describe your experience, try to frame it in ways that connect to their perspective. For example:

Instead of saying:

"Sometimes I just feel awful after meals."

Try saying:

"Within 30–60 minutes after eating, I often experience flushing, nausea, and diarrhea. This happens three to four times a week. Taking famotidine seems to lessen the severity."

This doesn't mean you need to "perform" for your doctor—it just makes it easier for them to see the medical relevance.

Sharing Responses to Treatment

Equally important is letting your doctor know how you respond to medications or interventions. If a drug helps, but only partly, note that. If it causes side effects, write that down. Over time, this feedback helps shape your treatment plan.

Creating a Long-Term Medical Management Plan

MCAS isn't usually something you fix overnight. For most people, it's an ongoing process of finding stability, learning their system, and adjusting as things change. That's why creating a long-term plan with your healthcare team is so important.

Step 1: Establish a Baseline

The first step is getting clear on where you are right now. Take time to identify your most disruptive symptoms—the ones that affect your daily life the most. Make a list of the treatments, medications, or lifestyle adjustments you're already using, and notice which ones seem to bring even small improvements and which ones don't seem to help at all. Writing this down can be eye-opening because it gives you a clearer picture of patterns you might not notice day-to-day. This personal baseline becomes the foundation for making thoughtful changes and, just as importantly, for tracking your progress over time.

Step 2: Prioritize Interventions

Because MCAS can affect so many parts of the body, the range of possible treatments can seem extensive and hard to sort through. That's why a good plan doesn't try to tackle everything at once—it prioritizes. For example, you and your doctor might decide to start by easing digestive symptoms with H2 blockers, and then, once those are better managed, add in mast cell stabilizers to help reduce overall flare activity. Breaking it down into clear, manageable steps makes the process more straightforward and allows you to notice improvements along the way.

Step 3: Build in Flexibility

MCAS isn't static—it can change with seasons, stress levels, hormones, or other health conditions. Your plan should be flexible. Instead of one rigid prescription, think of it as a "menu" of options you and your doctor can adjust.

For example:

- **Every day plan:** Baseline meds and lifestyle strategies.
- **Flare plan:** Extra medications or interventions for when symptoms spike.
- **Emergency plan:** Clear instructions for when to use epinephrine or seek

urgent care.

Step 4: Collaborate Across Providers

If you're working with multiple doctors, it's important to keep them connected, since each one may only see a small piece of your overall picture. Share your current medication list, any recent test results, and major updates across all your providers so that everyone stays on the same page. Even something as simple as creating a one-page summary letter—with your diagnosis, main symptoms, current treatments, and recent changes—can save time in appointments and prevent confusion or overlapping prescriptions. Some people even keep a small folder or digital file they can bring to each visit, which helps new doctors quickly understand their history without repeating the same story repeatedly. This not only makes your care safer but also helps you feel more in control of your treatment journey.

Step 5: Review and Adjust Regularly

Your plan is meant to grow and evolve with you, not stay frozen in place. Symptoms can shift, new treatments may become available, and your priorities might change over time. That's why it's helpful to build in regular check-ins—every 3 to 6 months—with your main provider. These appointments give you and your doctor a chance to review what's working, fine-tune your goals, and adjust your approach if needed. Think of it as keeping the plan flexible, so it always reflects where you are right now rather than where you were months ago.

Key Takeaways

- Finding the right doctor may take time, but pay attention to whether they listen and collaborate.
- Tracking what you feel—and what sets it off—is one of the most effective tools in your care.

- Clear communication—framing your experiences in ways that connect with medical thinking—helps you get better support.
- A long-term plan isn't just about prescriptions; it's about creating flexible strategies for everyday life, flare days, and emergencies.
- Remember: your voice matters. You are the expert on your own body.

2.4 Risks, Limitations, and Future Directions

When you're living with Mast Cell Activation Syndrome, it's natural to want clear answers and guaranteed solutions. If your system feels unpredictable, the thought of something solid to hold onto can be incredibly comforting. But the truth is, MCAS doesn't always fit neatly into medical boxes. Treatments that work beautifully for one person may barely make a dent for another. Some approaches carry risks, others are limited by a lack of research, and many questions about this condition still don't have simple answers.

That might sound discouraging at first—but it doesn't have to be. Understanding the risks and limitations is not about taking away hope. Instead, it's about giving you a realistic framework so you can make informed choices, protect yourself, and keep your expectations balanced. At the same time, there are exciting future directions—new therapies being studied, growing awareness in the medical community, and research that promises to shed light on what's really happening inside the body of someone with MCAS.

This section is about striking that balance: holding both honesty and hope.

The Risks: What to Be Aware Of

When we talk about "risks," we're not only referring to potential side effects from medications (though those are certainly important). Risks can also show up in other forms—like the emotional toll of getting your hopes up about a treatment that doesn't work, or the stress of navigating constant trial and error. There may also be financial risks, since many therapies aren't covered by insurance and costs can quickly add up. And sometimes the physical strain of testing new options can itself lead to setbacks before progress is made.

Recognizing the different dimensions of risk helps you approach decisions with clearer expectations and better support.

1. Medication Side Effects

Every medication used for MCAS has the potential to cause unwanted reactions. While many people tolerate antihistamines or mast cell stabilizers quite well, others find they trigger fatigue, high resting heart rate, dizziness, or even a paradoxical worsening of symptoms. Corticosteroids, for example, can be powerful tools in a flare, but long-term use carries serious risks like bone loss, immune suppression, and hormonal imbalance. (1).

2. Overlapping Conditions

Another risk in treating MCAS is the tendency for symptoms to overlap with other conditions. For example, fatigue, brain fog, and digestive upset could stem from mast cell activity—or they could be related to thyroid dysfunction, anemia, or even untreated sleep apnea. The danger is in attributing *everything* to MCAS and missing other treatable problems.

Doctors who are cautious and thorough will usually want to rule out these possibilities. While it can feel like extra hoops to jump through, this careful approach can actually save time and suffering in the long run.

3. Emotional Burnout

Searching for the perfect treatment plan can be exhausting. Those living with MCAS often describe feeling like a science experiment—constantly testing new supplements, rotating medications, and chasing protocols they've read about online. While curiosity, persistence, and self-advocacy are valuable strengths, this constant trial-and-error approach can take a heavy emotional toll, leading to frustration, burnout, and sometimes even a sense of discouragement. Recognizing this risk allows you to pace yourself, celebrate small victories, and focus on steady, sustainable progress rather than chasing perfection.

4. Financial Risks

Treatments can get expensive, especially if you're exploring beyond those treatments covered by insurance. Compounded medications, specialty supplements, integrative care visits, and experimental therapies can add up quickly. It's easy to feel pressured into trying "just one more thing." But not every option is worth the financial strain—especially if it hasn't been studied well.

Creating a budget (and sticking to it) can be as much a part of your care plan as tracking symptoms.

The Limitations: Where We Are Right Now

Research on MCAS is still in its early stages. Compared to well-studied conditions like diabetes or asthma, there are many unanswered questions about triggers, treatments, and long-term outcomes. Understanding these limitations doesn't mean giving up or settling for less—it means approaching management with both realism and hope. It's about making informed choices based on the knowledge currently available, while staying open to new discoveries, evolving protocols, and breakthroughs that may provide more clarity and options in the future.

1. Lack of Universal Testing Standards

One of the biggest limitations is in diagnosis. As we discussed earlier, lab tests like tryptase or urinary histamine can help, but they're not foolproof. Results can look "normal" even when someone is clearly having symptoms. That makes diagnosis slower and sometimes less certain.

This limitation can be incredibly frustrating for patients who are seeking medical validation. The silver lining is that awareness is growing, and researchers are actively exploring better biomarkers.

2. Inconsistent Medical Training

Because MCAS is relatively new on the medical scene, many providers simply haven't learned about it in training. This leads to wide variation in care: one doctor may be knowledgeable and supportive, while another may dismiss the condition altogether.

This inconsistency forces patients to become educators and advocates, which can feel unfair. But it also highlights the importance of resources like patient networks, advocacy groups, and medical conferences exploring emerging conditions and research.

3. One-Size-Doesn't-Fit-All

MCAS doesn't behave the same way in every body. One person may have skin-dominant symptoms, another may struggle most with their gut, and another may deal primarily with neurological or cardiovascular flares. This makes universal treatment protocols nearly impossible.

Instead, treatment remains highly individualized. The limitation here is that it takes time—and patience—to find what works for you.

4. Limited Research on Long-Term Outcomes

We don't yet have large, long-term studies tracking people with MCAS over decades. That means we don't fully understand how the condition evolves, what the most effective treatment combinations are, or whether certain approaches prevent progression. This doesn't mean no one is looking—it just means the evidence base is still growing.

On the Horizon: Expanding Understanding and Care

Here's the part that balances the picture: while risks and limitations are real, the future holds real potential. Each year, new studies, case reports, and clinical trials add to our understanding of mast cells and their role in health.

Advances in genetics, immunology, and precision medicine are also helping researchers connect the dots between MCAS and related conditions. This growing body of knowledge doesn't just expand treatment possibilities—it also increases awareness among healthcare providers, paving the way for earlier recognition, more accurate testing, and more individualized care.

1. Better Diagnostics

Researchers are working on identifying more reliable biomarkers for mast cell activation. Imagine a future where a simple blood draw or saliva test could clearly confirm MCAS without the uncertainty that patients face today. That's the direction many labs are moving toward.

2. Biologic Therapies

Biologics, like omalizumab (Xolair), are already being explored in MCAS. These medications target specific immune pathways and may one day offer a more precise way to calm mast cell overactivity without the blanket suppression of corticosteroids. Clinical trials are still small, but early results are promising.

3. Personalized Medicine

The future of MCAS treatment is likely to be deeply personalized. Instead of trial and error with long lists of medications, doctors may one day use genetic testing, immune profiling, and biomarker mapping to craft individualized plans. In other words: care tailored to your unique biology, not just how you feel.

4. Growing Awareness and Advocacy

Every year, more doctors, researchers, and patient groups are talking about MCAS. Conferences are being held, awareness days are spreading on social media, and new organizations are forming to support patients. While progress can feel slow, the momentum is building.

Living in the "In-Between"

Perhaps the most difficult part of dealing with risks, limitations, and future directions is learning to live in the "in-between." You're managing symptoms with the tools available now, while waiting for better answers on the horizon. That tension—between the reality of today and the promise of tomorrow—can be tough to hold.

Here's the encouragement: you don't have to do it perfectly. You don't have to chase every new treatment or have every answer figured out. It's enough to keep showing up for yourself, making thoughtful choices, and trusting that progress is happening, even if it feels slow.

Key Takeaways

- MCAS treatment involves learning to balance options while keeping an eye on side effects, emotional well-being, and financial sustainability.
- Research is still developing, but each year brings clearer testing methods, greater medical awareness, and more personalized approaches to care.
- The outlook is promising, with new diagnostics, targeted biologics, and innovative therapies being explored.
- Advocacy and awareness continue to grow, creating stronger support networks and better resources for those starting their journey.
- Living with MCAS means navigating today with resilience while remaining open to the expanding possibilities of tomorrow.

"When you help someone up a hill, you get closer to the top yourself."
– Norman Schwarzkopf

Let's make living with MCAS a little easier—together.
If this book is helping you understand your body, calm a flare, or feel more in control, please take a moment to leave a short review—it truly helps others find their way, too.

Help someone else find answers faster.
Remind another reader they're not alone.
Keep this book visible for those who need it most.

Thank you for being part of this growing circle of understanding and support—helping more people live steadier, better lives, one story at a time.

With gratitude,
Kathleen Dodwell

Follow the link or scan the code to leave your review -
https://mybook.to/jBGj

Natural Therapies and Lifestyle Strategies

Medication can play a crucial role—but it's often only part of the picture. Many people find that the day-to-day choices they make—what they eat, how they rest, the environments they spend time in—can either calm their system or stir it up. Natural therapies and lifestyle strategies may not be a cure, but they can provide your system with a gentler foundation, so it doesn't have to work quite as hard. This chapter explores practical, real-life adjustments that may help you feel steadier, including diet and supplements, stress relief, sleep habits, and pacing yourself. Think of this as your toolbox for building resilience—small, sustainable shifts that, over time, can make a big difference in how you feel.

3.1 Dietary Approaches

Food is one of the most basic human needs, and it's also one of the deepest sources of comfort and joy. We gather around meals to celebrate, to nurture each other, to slow down at the end of a long day. But when you live with MCAS, food can become complicated—sometimes even scary. Suddenly, the thing that once felt nourishing and normal may turn into a source of anxiety: *Will this meal trigger me? Will my body react this time, even if it didn't yesterday?*

If you've ever felt nervous staring at a plate of food, or found yourself googling ingredients before every bite, you're not alone. Lots of people with MCAS describe the same rollercoaster. Some days it feels like you've finally cracked the code—then the next day, a trusted food backfires. It's exhausting. And yet, food also holds one of the most powerful keys to calming mast cells and reclaiming stability. Learning how to work with your system instead of against it can open the door to more freedom, more confidence, and even more joy at the table again.

This section is about helping you understand the role diet plays in MCAS, and then giving you flexible tools to figure out what works for *you*. There is no single "MCAS diet." What soothes one person might trigger another. That's frustrating, yes—but it's also empowering once you realize you have permission to experiment and build a way of eating that's uniquely yours.

Let's explore the main dietary approaches people use, and more importantly, how you can use them in a way that feels supportive rather than restrictive.

The Low-Histamine Diet: A Starting Point, Not a Life Sentence

The basis of this approach is about reducing foods that are naturally high in histamine or that encourage your system to release histamine. The idea is simple: if mast cells are already misfiring, lowering the "histamine load" can give them less fuel to overreact.

But in practice, the low-histamine diet can feel overwhelming. The food lists are long and sometimes contradictory. One chart says you can eat spinach, another says avoid it. Some guides list strawberries as "okay in moderation," while others put them on the "never" list. It can leave you staring at your grocery cart, wondering, *What on earth is left to eat?*

Here's where it helps to reframe: the low-histamine diet is not meant to be a forever diet. Think of it as a reset button—a temporary way to lower the background noise in your system so you can hear the signals more clearly. By cutting back on the biggest histamine offenders for a few weeks, many people find their bodies calm down enough to start identifying which foods are actually a problem and which ones might be unfairly blamed.

Common High-Histamine Foods

The usual suspects include:

- Aged cheeses and cured meats
- Fermented foods (like sauerkraut, soy sauce, kombucha, yogurt)
- Alcohol, especially wine and beer
- Canned, smoked, or leftover fish and meats
- Tomatoes, spinach, eggplant
- Strawberries, citrus fruits, bananas
- Vinegar and vinegar-containing foods

But it's not just about "what" you eat—it's also about how fresh it is. Histamine levels climb as food sits, so leftovers, slow-cooked stews, or meat that's been thawed for days may trigger reactions even if the food itself isn't high-histamine. (1).

Elimination Diets: Playing Detective with Your Plate

An elimination diet is like playing detective. You remove potential suspects for a period of time, then reintroduce them one by one to see who's guilty.

This process can be tedious, but it's also one of the most powerful ways to uncover your unique triggers. And here's the good news: it doesn't have to be as extreme as some guides suggest. You don't need to cut out 90% of foods and live on rice and chicken forever. A thoughtful elimination plan involves making targeted, short-term changes and then listening carefully to your system's response.

How to Do It Without Losing Your Sanity

1. **Choose a clear starting point.** Many people start with the low-histamine framework and then remove other common culprits (like gluten, dairy, soy, or caffeine) if symptoms persist.

2. **Set a time frame.** Most eliminations last 2–4 weeks before testing reintroductions. Longer isn't better—your system needs variety and nourishment.
3. **Track your experience.** A simple journal noting what you ate, how you felt, and any flares can reveal patterns you might otherwise miss.
4. **Reintroduce one food at a time.** Go slowly—try one serving a day for a few days, and watch for reactions before moving to the next.

Nutritional Support: Feeding Your Mast Cells Well

Beyond avoiding triggers, diet can also play a role in stabilizing mast cells and supporting your overall health. Think of this as shifting from a mindset of restriction to one of nourishment. It's not only about what to take away—it's about what to add in.

Some nutrients and natural compounds have been studied for their ability to calm mast cells or reduce inflammation:

- **Vitamin C** – Acts as a natural antihistamine and mast cell stabilizer. (2). Foods rich in vitamin C (if tolerated) include bell peppers, kiwi, and broccoli.
- **Magnesium** – Supports relaxation of muscles and the nervous system, potentially calming reactivity. Found in pumpkin seeds, leafy greens, and certain mineral waters.
- **Bioflavonoids (like quercetin, rutin, luteolin)** – Plant compounds with mast cell-stabilizing properties. Found in apples, onions, and capers.
- **Omega-3 fatty acids** – Anti-inflammatory fats found in fish (if tolerated), flaxseeds, and chia seeds.

Some people choose to use supplements to ensure they're getting enough of these nutrients, especially if food options are limited. But whenever possible, whole foods are often gentler on the system and provide a broader range of benefits.

Practical Tips for Making Food Work in Real Life

Batch Cooking with Care

Leftovers can be tricky with MCAS, since histamine levels tend to rise the longer food sits in the fridge. But that doesn't mean you need to cook from scratch every single time you eat. A helpful strategy is to portion and freeze meals right after cooking, which locks in freshness and slows histamine formation. Later, you can reheat those frozen portions and enjoy them as if they were freshly made. Some people even find it useful to batch cook larger quantities of safe foods, then store them in single-serving containers for quick, low-stress meals.

Building a Safe List

Keep a running list of foods you know you tolerate well, whether it's a simple protein, a certain fruit, or a favorite grain. Having this personal "safe list" can be a real anchor on difficult days when decision-making feels draining. Instead of stressing over what to eat, you can fall back on these staples with confidence, knowing they're less likely to trigger a reaction. Some people even keep their list posted on the fridge or saved in their phone so it's always handy when meal planning or grocery shopping.

Eating Out Without Panic

Restaurants can feel intimidating, especially when menus are full of unknowns. One way to ease the stress is to call ahead and ask a few simple, direct questions, such as, "Can you prepare plain grilled chicken without marinade?" or "Could vegetables be cooked in olive oil only?" Framing your requests in clear, specific terms not only helps the kitchen staff understand but also increases the likelihood of getting a safe meal. Over time, you may even find a few "go-to" restaurants where the staff know your needs and make dining out feel less like a risk and more like a treat.

Be Gentle with Yourself

There will inevitably be slip-ups. You might eat something you believed was safe, only to experience a reaction afterward. This doesn't mean you've failed—it means you've gained more insight into your system's unique responses. Each flare adds another piece to the puzzle, helping you refine your food choices and strategies for the future. Over time, these lessons can build confidence and make navigating meals feel less uncertain.

The Emotional Side of Eating with MCAS

Food isn't just fuel—it's memory, culture, and connection. Losing access to favorite dishes can feel like losing pieces of yourself. Those living with MCAS often grieve the foods they once loved or feel left out when they can't fully participate in social meals and celebrations.

It's important to honor that grief, while also leaving room for possibility. Over time, some individuals find that their diets expand again as their symptoms stabilize. What feels out of reach today may become manageable tomorrow. In the meantime, experimenting with creative substitutions and focusing on the foods you *can* enjoy can help bring back a sense of comfort and pleasure at the table.

Key Takeaway

Dietary changes for MCAS aren't about perfection or punishment. They're about creating a calmer baseline so your system can feel more at ease. Whether you use a low-histamine reset, an elimination plan, or targeted nutrients, the goal is the same: to give you back a sense of control and freedom with food. And while the process can be frustrating at times, remember—you're not alone. Many others have walked this path, finding not only relief but also a new, gentler relationship with eating.

3.2 Natural and Complementary Therapies

Navigating MCAS typically means combining medication with other supportive strategies. You may find that adding natural or complementary therapies creates another layer of support, filling in the gaps that prescriptions can't quite cover. Think of it like weaving a safety net—medications might be the strongest ropes, but herbs, supplements, and mind-body practices are the smaller threads that make the net whole. Without them, things slip through. With them, the net holds steady.

This section will explore herbal remedies, supplements, and mind-body strategies that can help calm mast cells, soothe the nervous system, and bring a sense of empowerment to the healing process. None of these are quick fixes, and not everything works for everyone. But many people with MCAS find that experimenting with these tools—slowly, carefully, and with guidance—opens up new possibilities for stability and relief.

Herbal Options with Mast Cell-Stabilizing Potential

Herbal medicine has been used for centuries to calm inflammation, strengthen resilience, and support balance in the body. In recent years, modern research has begun to explore these traditional remedies in a more systematic way, uncovering evidence that certain plant compounds may directly influence mast cell activity. Early findings suggest that some herbs can help reduce mediator release or ease downstream inflammation, offering gentle but meaningful support. While the science is still emerging, these natural options can be considered as part of a broader, individualized approach to MCAS management.

Quercetin

Quercetin is a plant flavonoid found in apples, onions, berries, and green tea. It has been described as a "natural antihistamine." Research suggests that quercetin can stabilize mast cells, reducing their tendency to release histamine and other inflammatory chemicals. (1). It's often taken as a supplement in capsule form. Some people also increase quercetin-rich foods in their diet.

Curcumin

Curcumin, the bright yellow compound in turmeric, is another powerful anti-inflammatory agent. It may help reduce overall inflammation and can support calming overactive mast cells. (2). Curcumin is most commonly taken as capsules or powders added to foods, like smoothies, soups, or sauces. Its absorption improves when combined with black pepper (which contains piperine) or healthy fats such as olive oil, avocado, or coconut oil. Starting with small amounts allows you to gauge how your system responds, and you can gradually increase the dose if it's well tolerated. It can sometimes irritate sensitive stomachs or interact with certain medications. Begin with low doses and observe how your digestive system reacts, and consider checking in with a healthcare professional to ensure it fits safely into your MCAS management plan.

Other Herbal Allies

- **Green tea extract (EGCG):** EGCG is a key compound in green tea with antioxidant properties that help protect cells from damage. It also has gentle mast cell–stabilizing effects, which may help reduce flare intensity over time. (3). Many people take it in capsule form, though drinking high-quality green tea can also provide benefits. Starting with lower doses is wise, as concentrated extracts can sometimes cause mild digestive upset.
- **Stinging nettle:** Traditionally used for allergies, stinging nettle can help reduce sneezing, itching, and other histamine-driven symptoms. It's commonly consumed as a tea, tincture, or capsule. For sensitive individuals, starting with a smaller dose or weaker tea is recommended to gauge tolerance.
- **Boswellia (frankincense extract):** Boswellia has long been used to

support joint and tissue health thanks to its anti-inflammatory properties. (4). For people with MCAS who experience joint pain or inflammation during flares, Boswellia may provide supportive relief. It's often available as capsules or tablets, and, as with all supplements, working with a healthcare provider helps ensure safe and effective use.

These herbs are not cures, but they can be allies—gentle supports that, when layered with other strategies, help bring the body back into balance.

Supplements

Supplements are often the bridge between food and medicine. They deliver nutrients in higher concentrations than diet alone can provide, making it possible to target specific gaps or weaknesses in mast cell regulation and overall immune balance. While food provides the foundation, supplements can act as reinforcements—giving your system an extra boost where it needs support most. For people with MCAS, this can mean reducing the frequency or intensity of flares, supporting energy levels, or helping stabilize reactions that feel unpredictable.

Vitamin C

Vitamin C isn't just for colds—it also plays a big role in mast cell stability. Research suggests that it can reduce histamine levels in the blood, support antioxidant defenses, and help calm the intensity of flares. (5). Because it's water-soluble and rapidly used by the body, steady intake can make a noticeable difference for some people living with MCAS.

Typically taken in divided doses throughout the day, since the body doesn't store vitamin C well. Buffered or liposomal forms are often preferred, as they can be gentler on sensitive stomachs and sometimes better absorbed.

Magnesium

Magnesium helps regulate the nervous system, supports muscle relaxation, and plays a role in controlling inflammation. People living with MCAS are sometimes low in magnesium because ongoing stress and restricted diets make it harder to get enough through food alone. Replenishing magnesium can make a meaningful difference in how the body responds to daily triggers.

- **Forms:** Magnesium glycinate or citrate are generally well absorbed. Topical magnesium—such as sprays, lotions, or Epsom salt baths—can provide a soothing alternative, especially for those with digestive sensitivities.
- **Why it matters:** Adequate magnesium levels support healthy vagal nerve activity, which encourages the body to shift out of a constant fight-or-flight state and into a calmer, more balanced mode. This not only benefits mast cell stability but can also improve sleep, reduce muscle tension, and ease stress-related symptoms.

Diamine oxidase

Diamine oxidase (DAO) is the enzyme responsible for breaking down histamine in the gut. Some people with MCAS or histamine intolerance produce too little DAO, which means histamine from foods lingers longer and triggers reactions. (6).

- **How it's used**: Taken before meals, DAO supplements can help reduce food-related flares.
- **Limitations**: It doesn't fix mast cell misfiring itself, but it can reduce the burden on the system.

Mind-Body Therapies

This is where natural therapies move beyond the pill bottle. Mast cells don't act in isolation—they're deeply connected to the nervous system. When the body is in a state of chronic stress or hyper-vigilance, mast cells are more likely to misfire. Mind-body therapies work by calming the nervous system, breaking the cycle of stress and reaction.

Brain Retraining

Symptoms don't just come from mast cells releasing chemicals—they also come from the nervous system interpreting every signal as a possible threat. Over time, the body becomes like a smoke alarm that goes off not just for a fire, but for burnt toast, steam from the shower, or even dust floating by. Brain retraining aims to reset that alarm system, teaching the brain to tell the difference between real danger and harmless triggers.

This doesn't mean how you feel is "all in your head." Far from it. It means that your brain and body are in constant conversation, and sometimes the brain amplifies the body's distress signals. By gently reshaping those patterns, you can turn down the volume on symptoms, even if the mast cells are still sensitive.

How It Works in Practice

Brain retraining programs often involve a mix of visualization, affirmations, movement, and redirecting attention. At first, it may feel awkward—like learning a new language. But with daily practice, people often find their system begins to calm.

A common exercise might look like this:

1. **Notice a symptom or flare starting.**
2. **Pause and redirect.** Instead of focusing on the symptom, shift your attention to something soothing—maybe a memory of a safe place, or a

phrase like *"My body knows how to calm itself."*

3. **Pair with a physical cue.** Some programs use a hand gesture or a small movement to anchor the new response in the body.
4. **Repeat consistently.** The repetition helps the nervous system learn a new default pathway.

Why It Helps

- **Lowers baseline stress hormones (cortisol, adrenaline):** When the nervous system is on constant alert, stress hormones stay elevated, which can make mast cells more reactive. Brain retraining techniques help the body shift into a calmer state, reducing the background "noise" that keeps symptoms flaring. Over time, this calmer baseline makes it easier for mast cells to stabilize.
- **Breaks the cycle of fear fueling symptoms:** Living with unpredictable symptoms can create a feedback loop—symptoms trigger fear, and fear makes symptoms worse. Brain retraining interrupts this loop by teaching the brain new patterns of response, helping people step out of the constant fight-or-flight cycle and into a place of steadier resilience.
- **Gives people a sense of agency, even during flares:** One of the hardest parts of MCAS is the feeling of being out of control. Brain retraining provides practical tools—like breathing techniques, visualization, or redirecting attention—that allow people to take active steps, even when symptoms appear. This shift from helplessness to action can be profoundly empowering.

Brain retraining doesn't work overnight. It's more like strengthening a muscle—you build it rep by rep. But for many, it creates a foundation of calmness that medication alone can't provide.

Vagal Toning Techniques

The vagus nerve runs from the brainstem down through the chest and abdomen, touching the heart, lungs, and digestive organs. It's like the body's main "calm down" switch.

When the vagus nerve is strong and active, the body can easily shift into "rest and digest" mode. When it's weak or underused, the body stays stuck in "fight-or-flight", making mast cells more reactive. Vagal toning techniques gently exercise this nerve, helping the body remember how to calm itself.

Everyday Practices for Vagal Toning

1. **Breathing Exercises** – The simplest and most powerful tool. Try inhaling through the nose for a count of four, then exhaling through the mouth for a count of six or eight. The longer exhale signals safety to the nervous system.
2. **Humming or Singing** – Vibrations stimulate the vagus nerve as it passes the throat. A soft hum, a favorite song, or even chanting "om" can shift the body into a calmer state.
3. **Splashing Cold Water on the Face** – Brief cold exposure activates the dive reflex, calming heart rate and nervous system activity.
4. **Gentle Yoga Poses** – Positions like child's pose, supported bridge, or legs-up-the-wall help relax the vagus nerve and encourage the body into rest mode.
5. **Laughter** – Genuine belly laughs stimulate the vagus nerve and lower stress hormones. Watching a funny show or sharing time with a friend can be medicine too.

Reflection: Building a Muscle of Calm

Think of vagal toning like going to the gym. One session won't change much—but daily practice strengthens the body's resilience. Over time, the "calm down" response becomes stronger, making it easier to recover from triggers.

Meditation, Yoga, and Breathing Practices

In addition to brain retraining and vagal toning, more traditional practices like meditation, yoga, and structured breathing can be invaluable. Each of these encourages the body to pause, reset, and strengthen resilience.

- **Meditation** – Simple mindfulness practices can reduce anxiety, slow heart rate, and calm mast cell activity. (7). Even five minutes of sitting quietly, focusing on the breath, can make a difference.
- **Yoga** – Gentle, restorative forms of yoga help stretch and calm the body without overexertion. They also encourage awareness of breath and body connection.
- **Breathing practices** – Techniques like box breathing (inhale 4, hold 4, exhale 4, hold 4) give the nervous system a predictable rhythm that fosters safety and calm.

Takeaway

Natural and complementary therapies don't replace medical care, but they do expand the toolkit. Herbs like quercetin, supplements like vitamin C and DAO, and practices like brain retraining and vagal toning create multiple entry points for healing. Each small practice—whether it's a capsule, a cup of tea, a daily breathing exercise, or a moment of laughter—adds to the foundation of stability.

Healing with MCAS isn't about one single answer. It's about layering supports, patiently experimenting, and noticing what helps. Over time, these layers weave into a stronger net—one that can hold you through the ups and downs, offering more moments of ease, steadiness, and hope.

3.3 Environmental and Lifestyle Modifications

After learning about natural and complementary therapies in the previous section, it is important to look at how your surroundings and habits influence MCAS. When you are living with MCAS, it can sometimes feel like the whole world is filled with hidden landmines—perfumes in the grocery store aisle, cleaning products at a friend's house, a poor night's sleep, or even a little too much exertion. Our environments and daily rhythms play a massive role in how steady or unpredictable our mast cells are. Learning to make small, intentional changes in surroundings and routines can make the difference between constant flare-ups and a life that feels more manageable.

This isn't about striving for perfection or wrapping yourself in bubble wrap—it's about stacking the odds in your favor. Each change you make, no matter how small, is like removing one pebble from an overflowing backpack. Alone, it might not change everything, but together, they really lighten the load.

Let's look at three big areas where lifestyle and environment matter most: reducing chemical exposures, supporting restorative sleep and stress management, and finding balanced ways to move your system without tipping into exhaustion. Stories, examples, and reflections are included to make the ideas more relatable—helping you to picture how these concepts might take shape in your daily life.

Reducing Chemical Exposures

People living with MCAS often describe what they call "mystery reactions" that seem to strike without warning—hives after walking through a department store, brain fog after pumping gas, or nausea after visiting a neighbor who had just cleaned with bleach. While these reactions can feel baffling at first, they are not random. Environmental chemicals—especially synthetic fragrances, harsh cleaners, and other everyday toxins—can act like persistent irritants to mast cells, keeping them in a state of heightened sensitivity. (1). Understanding this connection helps explain why symptoms sometimes flare in places that others might not think twice about.

Fragrance-Free Living

Fragrance sensitivity tends to be a hallmark of MCAS. Scented laundry detergents, air fresheners, candles, lotions, shampoos, perfumes—these may smell pleasant to some, but for sensitive bodies, they're chemical cocktails waiting to spark a reaction.

Start with your own home. Switch to fragrance-free detergents, unscented soaps, and natural personal care items. Even this one shift can cut down daily exposures dramatically.

Non-Toxic Cleaning

Conventional cleaners often contain harsh chemicals like ammonia, bleach, and formaldehyde-releasing agents. These can trigger mast cells directly through inhalation or skin contact. (2).

Vinegar, baking soda, castile soap, and microfiber cloths can handle most cleaning needs. There are also non-toxic brands that list every ingredient clearly.

If switching everything at once feels overwhelming, start with the products you use most often, like dish soap or surface sprays.

EMF Sensitivity Considerations

Some people with MCAS notice symptoms flare around Wi-Fi routers, cell phones, or prolonged computer use. While research on EMFs (electromagnetic fields) and mast cells is still emerging, sensitivity is very real for some individuals. (3).

Turn off Wi-Fi at night, keep your phone on airplane mode when not in use, and avoid keeping devices near your bed.

Creating a Safe Home Base

Creating a calm, supportive home environment can make a real difference in managing MCAS. While the outside world may be full of unpredictable triggers, having a safe, low-stimulus space at home gives your system a chance to rest, reset, and recover. Small changes can make a big difference: air purifiers to reduce airborne irritants, opening windows for fresh ventilation, choosing natural fabrics that are gentle on the skin, and decluttering to reduce visual and mental stress. Even simple touches—like soft lighting, soothing colors, or a favorite chair—can create a sense of calm that helps both the body and mind. Over time, these intentional adjustments turn your home into a space that supports stability, comfort, and resilience, giving you a solid foundation to face the world outside.

Beyond physical changes, the home environment can influence emotional well-being too. Having areas dedicated to rest, quiet, or gentle hobbies reinforces a sense of safety and control, which in turn can help reduce mast cell triggers caused by stress. When your surroundings feel supportive rather than taxing, your system and mind can recover more efficiently, making it easier to navigate the unpredictable challenges of MCAS with steadiness and confidence.

Sleep Optimization and Stress Management

Sleep isn't just "rest time." It's when your system resets, repairs, and recalibrates. Poor sleep can make everything worse: symptoms flare more easily, emotional resilience drops, and the body has less buffer against triggers. Likewise, chronic stress keeps mast cells on high alert and primed to overreact. Learning to support sleep and manage stress isn't optional; it's essential. Even small, repeatable habits such as a consistent bedtime, a simple wind-down, and a few minutes of breathing can noticeably steady your day to day.

Sleep Optimization

The Basics of Good Sleep Hygiene

- **Regular schedule**: Going to bed and waking up at the same time each day helps regulate your system's internal clock.
- **Cool, dark, quiet environment**: Mast cells are sensitive to disruption, so creating a calm sleep environment reduces wake-ups.
- **Digital sunset**: Blue light from screens interferes with melatonin, the hormone that signals sleep. Try dimming lights and putting devices away an hour before bed.

Supporting Sleep with Gentle Tools

- Herbal teas like chamomile or lemon balm can be soothing.
- Magnesium glycinate before bed can relax the body.
- White noise machines or fans can block disruptive sounds.

Stress Management

Stress and mast cells are deeply intertwined. When the body experiences stress, it releases cortisol and adrenaline—chemical signals that can directly trigger mast cells to release their mediators. (4). This means that chronic stress is like leaving the "on" switch pressed for inflammation, subtly influencing symptoms day after day. Learning to manage stress doesn't mean eliminating it completely—life will always have challenges—but it does mean giving the body tools to return to calm more quickly and reliably. Over time, practicing stress management can reduce the intensity and frequency of mast cell flares, improve sleep, and enhance overall resilience.

Everyday Stress Soothers

- **Mini breaks:** Even two minutes of deep, intentional breathing between tasks can help reset the nervous system, calm the heart rate, and signal to the body that it's safe to relax.

- **Nature time:** Spending a few moments outside, feeling the sun, walking on grass, or listening to birdsong can lower stress hormones, support emotional balance, and create a natural buffer against flares. (5).
- **Creative outlets:** Journaling, drawing, gentle crafts, or even cooking mindfully can move the nervous system out of fight-or-flight mode and into a state of flow. These small practices remind the body and mind that calm and safety are possible, even amid daily challenges.

By weaving these simple stress-soothing habits into daily life, the nervous system gradually learns that it doesn't need to stay on high alert all the time. This, in turn, helps mast cells stay more balanced, reduces symptom spikes, and fosters a greater sense of control over daily well-being.

Reframing Stress

Sometimes, it's not just the stress itself that affects the body, but the way stress is interpreted and experienced. Thinking of symptoms or reactions as "failures" or as personal shortcomings can amplify tension and make mast cells more reactive. Shifting the perspective to see symptoms as signals from the body—messages that something needs attention, rest, or adjustment—can reduce the emotional weight of flare-ups. This reframing helps create a sense of partnership with the body rather than conflict, making it easier to respond calmly and strategically to challenges. Over time, approaching stress and symptoms with curiosity instead of judgment can lessen overall reactivity, support emotional resilience, and give a greater sense of control over daily health.

Exercise and Pacing Strategies for Energy Conservation

Movement is a double-edged sword for people with MCAS. On one hand, exercise supports circulation, mood, and resilience. On the other hand, overexertion can trigger flares, leaving you more symptomatic than before.

The key is finding the sweet spot—gentle movement that supports health without overwhelming the body.

Listening to Your Body's Signals

The old fitness mantra "no pain, no gain" doesn't apply with MCAS. Pushing through fatigue or discomfort can often backfire, triggering flares or worsening symptoms. Instead, think of movement as a dialogue with your system: it offers subtle cues when it's ready for gentle activity and louder signals when it needs a pause. Gentle pacing, short walks, stretching, or restorative exercises can keep muscles and joints active without overstimulating mast cells. Over time, this mindful approach helps build stamina, maintain flexibility, and support overall well-being, all while respecting the body's unique rhythm.

Gentle Exercise Options

- **Walking**: A simple, low-impact option. Even five minutes at a time counts.
- **Stretching and yoga**: Helps maintain mobility and calm the nervous system.
- **Water exercise**: Swimming or gentle movement in water takes pressure off joints and can be soothing.
- **Strength training with light resistance**: Builds stability without taxing the cardiovascular system too much.

The Role of Pacing

Pacing means balancing activity with intentional rest, tuning into the body's energy signals rather than pushing through regardless of how you feel. Individuals living with MCAS often experience unpredictable fatigue, and pacing helps prevent the "boom-and-bust" cycle—periods of feeling energized, overexerting, and then crashing. By planning activities around energy levels, spacing out tasks, and allowing for recovery breaks, it's possible to maintain more consistent stamina, reduce flares, and gradually build resilience over time. Pacing isn't about doing less forever; it's about learning to work with the body's rhythm to make daily life more manageable and sustainable.

Use a timer to remind yourself to rest, even if you feel okay.

Movement as Medicine

The goal isn't to train for a marathon—it's to establish a gentle, sustainable rhythm of movement that supports energy, mood, and overall health. Exercise is not about pushing the body to its limits; it's about nourishing it in a way that feels manageable and restorative, like tending to a garden with care, giving just the right amount of attention and encouragement for steady growth.

Takeaway

Environmental and lifestyle modifications are some of the most powerful tools for living with MCAS. By reducing chemical exposures, you create a safe foundation for healing. By supporting restorative sleep and managing stress, you give your nervous system a chance to reset. And by pacing your energy and finding gentle ways to move, you strengthen your system without overwhelming it.

These shifts aren't about perfection or control—they're about building a life that feels kinder to your system. Each change is an act of compassion toward yourself, a way of saying, *"I deserve to live in a space that supports my healing."* Over time, these small acts add up, creating a lifestyle that not only avoids flares but also fosters resilience, peace, and the possibility of joy in daily life.

Living Well with MCAS – Creating Your Personal Action Plan

By the time you've arrived here, you've probably gathered a lot of information. You've read about what mast cells are, how MCAS can affect the body, what kinds of treatments are available, and the many ways lifestyle choices can shape your health. Maybe you're feeling hopeful because you finally have language for what you've been going through. Or maybe you're feeling overwhelmed, staring at a mountain of options and wondering, *"Where do I even start?"*

The earlier parts of this book were about understanding the "why" and "what" of MCAS, this chapter is about the "how." How do you take all this knowledge and actually apply it to your life in a way that feels feasible and sustainable? How do you create a plan that supports you without feeling like another burden? How do you move from constant crisis mode into a place where you can breathe, plan, and even dream again?

This condition is as unique as the people who live with it. For one person, the key might be carefully tailoring their diet; for another, it might be finding the right medication combination, or pacing their energy to prevent flares. Some people thrive when they create highly structured routines, while others do better when they leave space for flexibility and gentle experimentation. What matters most is that your plan fits *you*—your system, your values, your lifestyle, your priorities.

Creating a personal action plan doesn't mean writing out a rigid checklist and holding yourself to impossible standards. It's not about doing everything at once or getting it "perfect." Instead, think of it like building a supportive toolkit or weaving together a patchwork garden. Each piece you add—whether it's a medication, a new bedtime ritual, a way to track symptoms, or a supportive friend you can call when you're struggling—becomes part of a larger picture that keeps you warm, steady, and safe.

In this chapter, you'll find practical steps for shaping your plan: how to set priorities, how to track what's working and what isn't, how to build your care team, and how to create daily rhythms that honor both your health needs and your life outside of illness. We'll also explore something that often gets overlooked: how to keep joy and meaning at the center of your plan. Because the goal isn't just to survive MCAS—it's to live well with it.

And let's be honest: "living well" doesn't mean living without challenges. Flares may still happen, setbacks may still come, and there may be days when the last thing you want to do is think about action plans. That's normal. Living well with MCAS is less about eliminating every struggle and more about learning how to ride the waves with more tools, more confidence, and more support at your back.

Imagine standing in a cluttered room. At first, it feels overwhelming—too many objects, too much noise. But then you start small. You clear one corner. You add a chair you love, a lamp that gives you comfort. Gradually, the space feels lighter, calmer, more yours. That's what creating an action plan for MCAS is like. You don't change everything overnight. You start with one corner of your life, then another. Over time, those changes add up until you're standing in a space that feels less like chaos and more like home.

So, take a deep breath. You don't have to have it all figured out today. You don't have to do everything at once. What you *do* need is a starting point, a sense of direction, and the reassurance that you're not alone on this path. This chapter will walk with you through the process, helping you sketch out a personal roadmap that feels realistic, compassionate, and hopeful.

By the end, you'll not only have a plan for managing MCAS, but you'll also feel empowered to keep adjusting it as your needs evolve, celebrate your progress along the way, and trust yourself as the expert of your own body.

4.1 Understanding Prognosis and Long-Term Outcomes

Prognosis is one of the first questions people ask after diagnosis, and it's also one of the hardest to answer. MCAS is unpredictable, and each journey is deeply personal. While there are no guarantees, understanding the spectrum of recovery, learning to manage expectations, and examining examples of people who successfully live with MCAS can help you approach the future with hope, strategy, and self-compassion.

In this section, we'll explore what recovery or remission can look like, how to manage expectations around degrees of improvement versus cure, and share detailed stories of people who have found ways to live successfully with MCAS. Along the way, we'll highlight reflections, practical takeaways, and ways to apply these lessons to your own life. By the end, you'll see that while MCAS can be challenging, it doesn't have to define the limits of your life.

What Recovery or Remission Can Look Like

When most people hear the word "recovery," they imagine a life entirely free of symptoms—a return to normalcy. MCAS rarely follows such a linear path. Recovery or remission can take a variety of forms. Some people experience extended periods without flares, allowing them to engage fully in work, social activities, hobbies, or family life. Others notice more subtle improvements: fewer flare-ups, reduced symptom severity, improved sleep, or the ability to anticipate and manage triggers. Even small victories—like being able to prepare a meal, taking a short walk, or enjoying a quiet moment without a flare—are deeply significant.

Recovery is rarely a straight line. People often experience cycles of improvement and setbacks. While this can feel discouraging at first, viewing setbacks as feedback from your system can be transformative. Each flare provides information about your triggers, limits, and strategies, offering a chance to adjust and refine your approach. Over time, even modest improvements accumulate, creating a sense of stability and confidence that feels life-changing.

Recovery can also differ based on your specific symptoms. Someone primarily affected by skin issues may see improvements through topical treatments or dietary adjustments, while someone struggling mainly with fatigue or cognitive challenges might find pacing, sleep optimization, and gentle exercise more effective. Understanding what improvement looks like for you personally is crucial for shaping your expectations and guiding your plan.

It's important to remember that recovery is fluid. What feels like a significant victory early in your journey may later become routine, allowing you to set new goals. Recognizing and celebrating progress, no matter how incremental, builds resilience and confidence over time.

Managing Expectations: Degrees of Improvement vs. Cure

One of the most essential lessons for anyone navigating MCAS is learning to distinguish between *improvement* and *cure*. A complete cure—a life entirely free of symptoms—may not be achievable for everyone. That doesn't mean meaningful progress isn't possible. Managing expectations involves redefining success, valuing incremental gains, and practicing self-compassion in the face of setbacks.

Expecting perfection can be exhausting. Many people spend years chasing a "magic cure," cycling through diets, supplements, medications, and lifestyle adjustments with hope and disappointment. Each flare can feel like failure, reinforcing anxiety and frustration. Shifting focus from perfection to progress allows you to reclaim a sense of control and agency.

It's helpful to view progress in two categories: *quantitative* and *qualitative*. Quantitative improvements might include fewer or shorter flares, more consistent sleep, reduced pain, or improved energy. Qualitative improvements can involve increased confidence in your ability to plan around flares, better emotional resilience, more engagement with hobbies and social life, and a sense of control over daily routines. Both are valid and meaningful.

Expectations should evolve over time. Early objectives might focus on simply getting through a workday or completing household tasks. Later, priorities may expand to include hobbies, social activities, or physical pursuits. Recognizing that progress is an ongoing journey rather than a fixed destination is essential for maintaining hope and resilience.

Reflections and Practical Takeaways

- Recovery can take many forms: extended flare-free periods, reduced severity, or better management of triggers.
- Progress is often incremental; small wins accumulate into meaningful long-term improvement.
- Define success on your own terms: living well is about engagement and autonomy, not perfection.
- Expect non-linear improvement: setbacks are inevitable, but they provide guidance and learning opportunities.
- Track, reflect, and adjust: journaling, symptom logs, and pattern recognition empower self-awareness.
- Emotional and social support matter: community, friends, family, and peer networks are essential for long-term outcomes.
- Celebrate resilience: every day you navigate MCAS with intention and care is a victory.

Understanding prognosis in this way emphasizes agency, patience, and self-compassion. MCAS doesn't define your life. Recovery and improvement come in many forms, and success is measured not by the absence of symptoms but by the ability to navigate life effectively, embrace progress, and celebrate both large and small victories. Living successfully with MCAS is not only possible—it is happening every day.

4.2 Building Your Healthcare & Support Team

In the midst of this uncertainty, one of the most powerful resources you can cultivate is a strong, reliable support network—a team of people who understand your condition, help guide your care, and support you in daily life. This section explores how to build that team, including strategies for communicating effectively with medical professionals, personal relationships, and peer networks.

A well-rounded healthcare and support team doesn't just respond to symptoms—it creates a sense of stability, safety, and partnership. With the right people in your corner, you gain more than medical input; you gain encouragement, validation, and a framework for making thoughtful choices. These individuals become part of your foundation, helping you find balance, maintain perspective, and keep moving forward, even when MCAS feels especially challenging.

Role of Primary Care Providers, Specialists, Nutritionists, and Therapists

The first pillar of your support team is your healthcare providers. MCAS is multi-systemic and can require collaboration among several professionals. At the center of this network is your primary care provider (PCP). A PCP is not just the doctor you see once a year for checkups—they are your coordinator, advocate, and go-to source for navigating the complexity of your health. A skilled PCP monitors your overall health, manages medications, and coordinates referrals to specialists.

Specialists are often critical in MCAS management, tailored to your unique symptoms. Allergists, immunologists, gastroenterologists, cardiologists, neurologists, and dermatologists may all play important roles. For instance, someone with severe gastrointestinal issues might rely heavily on a gastroenterologist familiar with histamine intolerance and mast cell triggers, while someone experiencing cognitive challenges might benefit from a neurologist who understands MCAS-related brain fog and headaches. The key is finding specialists who are not only knowledgeable but willing to collaborate, listen, and respect your lived experience.

Guidance from a nutritionist or registered dietitian can be a key part of recovery. Diet plays a significant role in managing mast cell triggers, and a professional can help you navigate low-histamine, elimination, or other specialized diets safely and sustainably. Rather than imposing rigid rules, a supportive nutritionist works with you to identify triggers, maintain nutritional balance, and implement gradual adjustments that integrate into your life without creating unnecessary stress.

Therapists, including psychologists, counselors, and occupational therapists, provide vital support for the emotional and cognitive challenges of MCAS. Living with a chronic, unpredictable condition can create anxiety, depression, and stress that exacerbate physical symptoms. Therapists help develop coping strategies, mindfulness practices, pacing techniques, and stress-reduction tools. Occupational therapists, in particular, can offer practical solutions for energy conservation, ergonomic modifications, and activity planning, helping you create a sustainable daily routine.

It's important to remember: your healthcare team works best with you, not just for you. You are the expert in your own body, and your observations about triggers, symptoms, and effective strategies are invaluable. Open communication, careful record-keeping, and active collaboration can turn a fragmented approach into a cohesive, life-enhancing system.

Importance of Support Groups and Patient Advocacy Networks

While medical support is crucial, emotional and community support is equally important. MCAS can be isolating, especially because symptoms are often invisible. Friends, family, or colleagues may struggle to understand the challenges, leaving you feeling alone or misunderstood. Support groups and advocacy networks provide connection, validation, and practical guidance.

Support groups, whether in-person or online, allow you to meet people who understand the unpredictable nature of MCAS. Sharing experiences reduces isolation and provides actionable advice—everything from symptom management to coping strategies and dietary tips. Being part of a community where others "get it" can be profoundly reassuring and empowering.

Patient advocacy networks offer another layer of support, providing educational resources, connecting members to knowledgeable doctors, and advocating for broader awareness of MCAS. Engagement with these networks can give you purpose, a sense of belonging, and access to the latest research and therapies.

These networks also address challenges that medical professionals may not always consider, such as workplace accommodations, social pressures, and lifestyle adjustments. They create a safe space where you can ask questions, share setbacks, and celebrate successes without judgment.

Communicating with Family, Friends, and Workplace About MCAS

Even the best medical and community support won't feel complete if the people closest to you don't understand your needs. Clear, honest communication is essential for building a truly supportive environment.

Start with family and close friends. Take time to explain what MCAS is, how it shows up in your daily life, and what tends to trigger flares. Be candid about your limitations and needs—without apology. Help them recognize that fatigue, brain fog, or sensory sensitivity isn't laziness or avoidance; it's part of the condition. Sharing reliable resources, such as information from medical specialists, trusted websites, or patient advocacy groups, can also go a long way in helping loved ones grasp the reality of MCAS. Sometimes hearing it from a doctor or reading reputable materials makes the condition feel more concrete and easier to understand.

Small adjustments—like keeping social plans flexible, choosing low-trigger environments, or being mindful about foods and fragrances—can make an enormous difference. Over time, these conversations not only reduce misunderstandings but also help build a foundation of trust and mutual care.

Workplace communication is equally important. Advocating for accommodations such as flexible hours, remote work options, or scheduled breaks can greatly improve productivity and health. Framing your requests around maintaining performance and safety often resonates best with employers. Documentation from healthcare providers can support your requests, but clarity and professionalism go a long way in fostering understanding.

Being clear about your needs—and setting healthy boundaries—makes a big difference. You don't have to share every detail of your condition, but offering enough context helps others know how to support you. Friends don't need to see lab results, but they may appreciate knowing which foods or scents to avoid. In the workplace, managers don't need your full medical history, but they can be more supportive if they understand practical needs like flexible breaks or adjusted workloads.

Integrating Your Team Into a Cohesive Support System

Building a team is about creating a network that communicates, collaborates, and complements one another. Your PCP can coordinate care, but you remain the hub—tracking symptoms, observing patterns, and noting which interventions work.

A well-integrated team ensures that medical treatments, lifestyle strategies, and social support all align. For example, if your nutritionist recommends a dietary adjustment that affects medication absorption, communicating with your prescribing doctor prevents complications. If a therapist introduces pacing strategies, sharing them with your family ensures they understand why certain activities are limited.

Regular check-ins—through medical appointments, support groups, or personal reflections—keep the system dynamic and responsive. This collaborative network allows you to manage flares, pace energy, and support emotional well-being in a coordinated way.

Practical Takeaways for Building Your Team

- **Start with a primary care provider** who coordinates care and values your lived experience.
- **Identify specialists** based on your symptom profile and personal needs. Seek those willing to collaborate.
- **Engage nutritionists or dietitians** to guide safe, individualized dietary strategies.
- **Incorporate therapists** for emotional, cognitive, and practical support.
- **Join support groups and advocacy networks** for community, validation, and resources.
- **Communicate clearly with family and friends** about needs, triggers, and boundaries.
- **Advocate in the workplace** for accommodations that support health and productivity.
- **Maintain coordination** between all team members through logs, updates, and communication.
- **Take ownership of your journey**—your observations and experiences are critical.
- **Celebrate progress**—every day you navigate MCAS with intention is a victory.

A well-constructed healthcare and support team provides not only guidance for symptom management but also emotional reassurance, personal empowerment, and long-term stability. Each member—professional or personal—contributes to a web of understanding, trust, and collaboration, allowing you to live more confidently and intentionally with MCAS.

4.3 Creating Your Personalized Plan

A personalized plan gives you a compass when the path feels unclear—anchors to hold during the swells and a map to steer you toward calmer waters.

In this section, we'll walk through a step-by-step framework for shaping your plan. We'll talk about how to identify your triggers and track how you feel, how to experiment with medications or natural therapies, and how to layer in lifestyle changes without burning yourself out. Then, we'll explore how to adapt as things shift — because with MCAS, they will.

Step One: Identifying Triggers and Tracking Symptoms

Figuring out triggers can be complicated. At times, the connection is straightforward—"I ate that food, and then I reacted." Other times, the reaction seems to appear without any clear cause, making it difficult to predict or prevent.

That's why tracking is so powerful. Think of it as turning on a flashlight in a dark room. Without it, you're stumbling around, bumping into things, and feeling frustrated. With it, you start to see patterns you couldn't see before.

Why tracking matters

Our brains aren't designed to hold weeks of detailed health information. When symptoms are unpredictable, it's easy to lose track of connections. That's where a simple log or journal comes in — not as a homework assignment, but as a gift to your future self. By jotting down what you eat, what you're exposed to, how you feel, and any flares that happen, you create a record that helps you and your care team make sense of the chaos.

Making it achievable

The trick is not to overcomplicate things. Some people love color-coded spreadsheets and symptom-tracking apps; others prefer a notebook with a few quick notes. The "best" system is the one you'll actually stick with. Even something as simple as writing:

- Breakfast: oatmeal, blueberries
- Medications: morning antihistamine

- Activity: short walk, 20 minutes
- Symptoms: mild flushing, fatigue at 2 pm

That alone can reveal useful patterns over time.

Looking for patterns

After a few weeks, you may notice that certain foods, environments, or stressors often precede flares. Maybe it's red wine, scented laundry products, or lack of sleep. Other times, it's not one single trigger but a "bucket effect" — your system can handle some stressors, but once the bucket overflows, symptoms erupt. Seeing this in black and white can be validating and empowering.

Gentle reminders

Of course, tracking has its pitfalls. Some people become hyper-focused, turning every meal into an anxiety spiral. If you find yourself stressed by the process, step back. Remember, the goal is insight, not perfection. Track enough to see patterns, but not so much that it steals your peace.

Step Two: Selecting Medications and/or Natural Therapies to Try

Once you've identified your triggers, the next step is to work closely with your healthcare professionals to tailor safe choices that help steady your system—medications, natural supports, or a thoughtful mix. It can feel like facing an enormous menu, unsure what to pick. There isn't a single "best" treatment; what's transformative for one person may barely move the needle for another.

Starting small, going slow

One of the wisest approaches is the "start low and go slow" method. Think of your system as a sensitive tuning fork — if you slam it with too many changes at once, the vibrations get overwhelming. But if you introduce one change at a time, you can actually hear the notes and decide if they're helping.

Medications

Some people find relief with antihistamines (H1 and H2 blockers), mast cell stabilizers, or other supportive meds their doctors prescribe. These medications are not a cure, but a way to steady the ride while you learn to manage your condition.

Natural therapies

Other people supplement with natural options such as quercetin, vitamin C, magnesium, or gentle herbal supports. Again, the key is to try one at a time, at a low dose, and track your response. Natural doesn't always mean harmless — especially for sensitive bodies — so respect your limits.

Building your "toolbox"

Think of medications and natural therapies as tools in a toolbox. You may not need every tool every day, but when something breaks down, it's good to have the right wrench ready. Your plan doesn't need to be a single "magic bullet." It can be a combination of supports that, together, keep you steady.

The contents of this book are for informational purposes only and do not constitute medical advice; always consult a qualified healthcare professional before making any decisions about your health, medications, or treatment plan.

Step Three: Implementing Lifestyle Changes and Measuring Progress

With triggers better understood and tools starting to take shape, the next step is weaving changes into daily life. This is the stage where your plan shifts from theory to practice—where strategies move off the page and into real routines. It's about building patterns and habits that support stability, not just during flares but also in the steadier moments in between. Over time, these small, consistent adjustments create a stronger foundation for living more comfortably and confidently with MCAS.

One step at a time

The temptation is to overhaul everything at once — to start a new diet, a new exercise plan, a new sleep routine, and a new supplement all in the same week. But that's a recipe for burnout, so instead, think about adding one change, seeing how it settles, then layering in another.

Food and routine

Maybe your first step is adjusting your meals — swapping a few high-histamine foods for gentler ones. Or maybe it's focusing on sleep, creating a simple bedtime ritual with dim lights and calming music. Progress doesn't always mean big leaps. Sometimes it's as small as noticing that going to bed 30 minutes earlier helps you wake up with a little more energy.

Measuring progress

This is where the effort you've put into tracking really shows its value. Progress with MCAS is often subtle and easy to miss without a record. A symptom that once appeared daily may shift to only a few times a week, or a flare that used to last days might now resolve within hours. These gradual shifts are meaningful signs that your plan is helping your system move toward greater stability. Recognizing them not only builds confidence but also helps you and your healthcare team fine-tune your approach.

The balance of structure and flexibility

Your plan should give you enough structure to feel supported but enough flexibility to handle life's surprises. Too much rigidity can be like a prison; too much looseness can leave you adrift. Aim for a middle ground where your routines support you, not cage you.

Adapting the Plan Over Time

Even with the best planning, life with MCAS is rarely static. That's why your plan isn't a finished product — it's a living framework you'll keep reshaping as you go.

Thinking like a scientist

Approach your plan with curiosity. If something stops working, it doesn't mean you've lost progress. It means it's time to tweak the experiment. Maybe your bucket is fuller because of stress, or maybe a new environmental factor has crept in. Adjust, observe, and adapt.

Building resilience

Adapting also means building resilience — both physically and emotionally. When setbacks happen, remind yourself: this isn't the end of your progress. It's part of the process. Many people find that over time, even if flares still happen, they recover faster or handle them with more confidence. That's growth, too.

The long view

Over the years, your system can change, your understanding deepens, and your strategies expand. The plan you create today won't be the same one you use ten years from now — and that's a good thing. It means you're evolving with your condition, not against it.

Bringing It All Together

Creating your personalized plan for MCAS involves weaving together supports that allow you to live more fully within your reality. You start by shining a light on your triggers, experiment gently with therapies, and layer in lifestyle changes one by one. Over time, you track, adapt, and grow — not toward perfection, but toward a life that feels more manageable, more meaningful, and more yours.

Your plan is your garden and your compass. It won't look like anyone else's, and it doesn't have to. The most important part is that it gives you hope, steadiness, and a sense that you're no longer stumbling in the dark.

Like any good garden, your plan will keep changing with the seasons — but with steady care, it can grow into something nourishing and deeply your own.

Take heart: every step you take, no matter how small, is a seed planted. Over time, those seeds grow into something real and sustaining — a life with MCAS that is not just about surviving, but about living well.

How to Track Triggers - A Practical Guide

Grab the free trigger-tracking template below to get started.
Keep it as is, tweak it to fit your day,
or use it as inspiration to build your own.

Download here - ***http://bit.ly/4nj3Wtp***

Or scan the code

Ready to begin? Here's your step-by-step guide to tracking your triggers.

1) Pick one question to answer this month.

Examples: "Which foods tend to precede my afternoon flushing?" "What changes after a bad night's sleep?" "Do fragrances set me off?"

Write your question at the top of your log. It keeps you focused.

2) Choose the easiest way to write things down.

Download our free tracking spreadsheet, or use a Notebook, Notes app, simple document—whatever you'll actually use. Keep it where you'll see it (kitchen bench, bedside, phone home screen).

3) Use the same short headings every time.

Spend 30–60 seconds, 3–5 times a day. Use these headings and fill them in briefly:

- **Food & drink:** include if it was fresh or a leftover (and how old).
- **Meds & supplements:** name + dose + time.
- **Exposures:** fragrance, cleaning products, smoke, pets, pollen, travel, heat/cold.
- **Activity & stress:** movement, big stress, pacing changes.
- **Sleep:** hours + quality (good / fair / poor).
- **Symptoms or "yellow lights":** what you felt, when it started, how strong; what helped.

4) Add timing, not just "what."

Note *when* things happen in relation to anchors: meals, meds, and sleep.

Examples: "1 hr after lunch—face warmth," "woke 3 a.m.—palpitations," "30 min after perfume on train—itch."

5) Include amounts.

Portions and doses matter.

Examples: "½ glass red wine," "1 tsp cinnamon," "cetirizine 10 mg," "two spritzes perfume nearby."

6) Note freshness and prep.

Circle anything that you know raises histamine or sits around: leftovers (how many days), slow-cooked/fermented/aged foods, canned fish, very ripe fruit, reheated meals, restaurant meals (add brand/venue if useful).

7) Know your "baseline" and your early warnings.

First, write what a typical day looks like for you when things are "normal" (your **baseline**): usual symptoms (if any), energy, sleep, digestion, skin, etc.

Next, make a short list of your **early warning signs** ("yellow lights")—the first hints a flare might be starting, like itchy palms, face warmth, brain fog, or queasiness.

Whenever you notice one of these yellow lights, **note the time and what just happened** (meal, exposure, stress, heat). Catching these early cues helps you take action sooner.

8) Rate intensity.

Use a tiny scale and stick to it. Example: **0–3** (0 = none, 1 = mild, 2 = moderate, 3 = strong).

Write: "flushing 2/3; dizziness 1/3; hives 0/3." No essays needed.

9) Change just one thing at a time.

Testing a hunch? Make *one* change for 7–14 days (e.g., switch to unscented detergent **or** avoid leftovers). If you start a new med or supplement, note the date, dose, and any effects.

10) Do a 2-minute evening tidy.

Fill the gaps for anything you missed, then **circle** the biggest exposures or events. If you had a flare, **star** the 24 hours before it and note what happened during the next 6–8 hours—this window is gold for patterns.

11) Do a 15-minute weekly check.

Flip through the week and look for:

- **Same pairing repeats?** (e.g., leftovers → flushing within 1–2h)
- **Amount matters?** (a small serving is fine; a larger one triggers symptoms)
- **Timing window?** (symptoms show up 30–60 min after fragrance; next morning after poor sleep)
- **Bucket effect?** (several small stressors stack up on flare days)
- **What helped?** (things that consistently shorten or soften symptoms)

Then write 2–3 sentences:

"This week, likely triggers - ___. Yellow lights - ___. What helped - ___."

12) Choose one next step for the coming week.

Examples: "Avoid leftovers" "Take a 10-minute outdoor break after fragrance exposure," "Take evening H2 antihistamine earlier (per clinician)."
Write it at the top of next week's page.

Optional tweaks (use only if helpful)

- **Short tags beat long notes:** add 1–3 tags like #leftovers, #perfume, #poorSleep, #heat, #exercise.
- **Log around transitions, not all day:** wake, meals, meds, exercise, commute, bedtime.
- **Hormones/illness/weather:** add menstrual cycle day, infections, heat waves, storms, high pollen if they matter for you.
- **"Rule of 3" for patterns:** treat it as a pattern after you've seen the same pairing **three times** in similar timing windows; before that, call it a "maybe."

Common snags (and fixes)

- **Tracking is stressing me out.** Just note meals, meds, sleep, and symptoms. It's okay to log less on quiet days.
- **I decided X is "the" trigger after one event.** Don't do that, wait for the **rule of 3** and check timing windows.
- **I changed three things and can't tell what worked.** Reset; change one variable per week.
- **I missed a day.** No problem—pick it up tonight. Progress > perfection.

What success looks like

- You can name your top 2–3 likely triggers and the timing window that links them to reactions.
- You recognize your yellow lights early and have a short calm-down routine

you use automatically.

- Your notes make appointments easier—you and your clinician see the pattern at a glance and decide faster, with more confidence.
- You're logging less but learning more—brief entries still reveal clear patterns.
- Over a few weeks, you notice fewer surprises (or milder flares) and more steady days.

Bottom line: keep it short, keep it steady, and let the patterns do the talking.

Patient Stories

Lena's Story:

Lena was forty-one when life narrowed to the size of a living room couch. Previously, she had been a stay-at-home mum who moved through a house full of small feet and noisily ordinary chaos—school lunches, soccer practices, whispered bedtime stories. Her world revolved around caregiving: wake, feed, ferry, soothe. It was whole in the way that only family life can be.

Then, slowly and for no obvious reason, things changed. Fatigue set in, heavy and unrelenting. At first, Lena thought she just needed a long weekend or a bit more sleep, and that it would pass. But the tiredness stayed. Days blurred together with a deep exhaustion that naps couldn't fix. Brain fog became a regular part of her life. Words slipped away mid-sentence, recipes went wrong, and managing the household started to feel impossible.

Doctors labeled it post-viral fatigue and, eventually, Myalgic Encephalom yelitis/Chronic Fatigue Syndrome (ME/CFS). The diagnosis explained some things. It also felt like a verdict: a slowly closing door on the active, engaged life she'd known. Lena learned to conserve energy, to ration herself in a way that felt humiliating but necessary. Friends dropped by less often once they noticed she couldn't always keep plans. Her identity as a mother and a doer was quietly reshaped into someone who measured activity in spoons and planned small victories.

For years, that was her reality. Then new symptoms appeared, at first seeming unrelated but impossible to ignore. Her skin itched in waves. Her pulse fluttered without warning. She began to have intense digestive flares: cramping, diarrhea, and nausea after meals or even hours later. The gut problems didn't stay isolated. When her stomach acted up, everything else got worse. Brain fog became so thick she could barely read, fatigue deepened, dizziness returned, and her muscles ached all over. It felt like her gut controlled everything, and when it acted up, her whole body crashed.

Lena felt like she was living in a body that had taken on its own weather system—clear skies one morning, full storms the next. The unpredictability was the worst part. Grocery shopping became a trial: would lunch trigger a three-day slump? Would a simple dinner derail the next week? She tried to explain to her partner, to friends, but words failed. "You look fine," people would say, and those words landed like blows. There were nights she cried quietly, not just from pain but from a grief she couldn't name—the loss of things she'd always taken for granted: spontaneous outings, the stamina to play on the floor with her kids, the ability to plan without fear.

Over time, patterns emerged. Lena became a meticulous tracker. She wrote down meals, the timing of symptoms, sleep length, stressors, medications—anything she could think might be relevant. The journal was both a lifeline and a torment; it showed patterns but also reminded her how little control she seemed to have. In those pages, one pattern screamed louder than the rest: when the gut flared, everything else did too. Digestive distress seemed to be the headline, summoning a troop of other symptoms in its wake.

Her primary care doctor was helpful at first, offering advice on symptom management, sleep, and gentle encouragement. But things changed when Lena brought up Mast Cell Activation Syndrome. She had learned about it from patient forums and support groups, where people described symptoms much like hers: flares affecting many systems, reactions to foods and fragrances, and a strong link between gut issues and crashes. Her doctor was cautious. "It's not well understood," she said. "We can try antihistamines and see if they help."

They tried. H1 and H2 antihistamines brought some relief, with less itching and fewer waves of flushing, but the digestive problems continued. Mast cell stabilizers were also tried; some helped a bit, while others caused side effects that felt worse than the illness itself. Lena went through different medications and supplements with steady but tired determination: cromolyn made her bloated, quercetin upset her stomach, and probiotics sometimes helped but sometimes didn't. Each new attempt brought hope, followed by disappointment.

Worse than the medications that failed was losing trust in her own body. She started to think that every mistake—every slip in her diet or missed nap—was her fault. Tasks that used to be easy now felt like battles she had to win with herself. This constant struggle fed a quiet, ongoing anxiety that made recovery seem always out of reach.

There were moments of acute despair. Lena remembers a winter when the kids came home from school with colds, and the household's minor illnesses turned into a prolonged storm for her. Her stomach refused food for days, and when she did eat, the pain was volcanic. She slept in short fits and woke more exhausted than before. Friends suggested she try another diet, a cleanse, a new supplement—"You have to try everything," someone urged—but she had already tried so much. She felt like a case file rather than a person; every new suggestion was a test she had to pass or fail. It felt endless, and at times she thought life had narrowed to merely surviving episodes.

Then, by a combination of persistence and benign luck, Lena found a clinician with a different approach. This doctor listened. She had experience with complex immune dysregulation and an openness to therapies that weren't mainstream. She explained carefully: while standard treatments were first-line and important, some patients with severe, gut-centered MCAS had benefited from judicious use of peptides—short chains of amino acids that can modulate immune and tissue-repair pathways. The explanation was careful, not miraculous. "These are off-label uses," the doctor said. "Not magic. But for some people, they help stabilize the gut in a way other treatments have not."

Lena listened, suspicious but desperate in equal measure. The word "peptide" sounded clinical and alien, and she worried about chasing another long list of pills without clear returns. Still, the pattern in her life was undeniable: when her gut calmed, everything calmed. If there were even a chance to quiet that central switch, she wanted to try.

The protocol began slowly and conservatively. The clinician ordered baseline labs, reviewed potential interactions, and set expectations: there might be flares, and results could take weeks to months. They started with a peptide aimed at supporting mucosal healing and immune modulation. Lena's first weeks were a mixture of vigilance and guarded hope. She kept the journal, careful to note any shifts.

Small changes came first. Lena had nights with less waking and mornings when brain fog felt lighter, more like a thin veil than a wall. The first month wasn't life-changing, but she noticed a new sense of lightness. By the second month, she had fewer severe gut flares. Meals still took planning, but the worst breakdowns became less common. As her gut calmed, her brain fog eased, pain lessened, and dizziness happened less often. The changes weren't instant or perfect, but they were clear in her daily life.

Relief came at a price. The peptides were an off-label therapy and expensive. Insurance didn't cover them, so the financial strain added to the stress of an already tough situation. Lena and her partner adjusted their budget, made sacrifices, and relied on family for help. The trade-offs were real, but the benefits—like being able to bathe the kids without needing to rest afterward, or reading a story without losing her place—were worth it.

As months went by, Lena adjusted to a new normal. The peptide treatment became part of a bigger plan: regular H1 and H2 antihistamines, mast cell stabilizers as needed, a simple gut-friendly diet, careful food handling to avoid histamine build-up by choosing fresh or frozen meals, and nervous system practices like short meditations and paced rest to prevent energy crashes. The peptides helped her gut heal and resist flares, while the other steps supported her overall health.

The change in her mindset was significant. For years, every meal felt like a battle, and every social event was a risk. Once her gut calmed, that constant tension faded. Lena started planning again. She brought back safe activities, like attending a short school play, having a picnic with carefully prepared food, or spending a morning at the park that ended with happy, tired kids instead of exhaustion. At first, the freedom was subtle, just a sense that her home didn't have to feel like a hospital. Soon, it grew into bigger joys. She began volunteering at the school library once a week, a small role that let her be present without overdoing it. She enjoyed cooking safe meals for her family and watching them eat without worry.

Her relationship with her partner deepened under the strain and the recovery. They learned to communicate better about limits and needs. He took on more grocery runs and morning routines when she felt fragile. He learned to see the progress in small increments: fewer urgent calls to the bedroom, more evenings with laughter rather than exhaustion. Lena's children, who had grown used to a quieter version of their mother, began to see her return—not to the woman she had been before illness, but to a version who could show up in meaningful ways again.

There was also a community element to her recovery. Lena still attended a support group for people with ME/CFS and MCAS. There, she found people who understood the particular terror of a gut flare and the slow victory of a good week. She shared resources—a podcast episode on peptides here, a practical tip on freezing single-serve meals there—and, in return, received the steady validation that scientific progress is often incremental and messy.

Even now, Lena's life has boundaries. She still avoids some restaurants. She still plans recovery time after social events. She remains cautious about new supplements or treatments. But the tenor of her days changed from one dominated by dread to one that includes cautious hope. Where she once worried she might never again play actively with her children, she now builds forts on the living room floor and reads books aloud without drifting in and out of coherence. The victories are not dramatic headlines, but they are life-sized and true.

When people ask what made the difference for her, Lena answers honestly and with nuance. The peptides were a turning point—an intervention that finally allowed her gut to stop firing so wildly and, by doing so, gave the rest of her system room to stabilize. But she is careful to add what the clinician emphasized at the outset: these therapies are not universal cures. They work in some people and not in others, and they must be used thoughtfully, with medical oversight and realistic expectations. For Lena, the peptides unlocked a path forward; for someone else, they might be ineffective or inadvisable.

Her final piece of counsel is tender and practical: measure progress in what actually matters. For her, that meant counting the days when she could make dinner, the afternoons when she could sit through a school event, the evenings when she could be present and not merely surviving. In the long ledger of illness and care, those small, repeated wins are what add up.

Lena's story isn't a simple tale of success. It's filled with tough choices—financial, emotional, and physical—and times when progress stalled and hope faded. But it's also a story of recovery built on careful listening, medical curiosity, and an approach that fits her body's needs. Her gut had been the biggest challenge in her life, but as it quieted, the rest of her life slowly returned.

James's Story:

James was forty-nine, a father of three, and a project manager in the construction industry. Before COVID, his life was full—long hours on job sites, weekend bike rides with friends, and noisy family dinners where his kids swapped stories across the table. He had always been the steady one, the reliable anchor. If a pipe burst, he found the shut-off valve. If the schedule slipped, he recalibrated. If a kid forgot a science project, he was the one at the kitchen bench with cardboard and glue at 10 p.m. So when he caught COVID in late 2020, he assumed he'd bounce back quickly. He didn't.

At first, the lingering cough and fatigue seemed like just an inconvenience. He tried to walk it off with short loops around the block and a slow jog, determined to prove he still could. Weeks went by, but the cough never really faded. Climbing stairs left him breathless, his chest tight, as if a strap was pulled around his ribs. Even short walks made his heart pound and his pulse race more than usual. He thought it was just post-viral recovery and told himself to give it time. But the symptoms didn't go away; they only grew. His nose ran constantly in certain places, and even a hint of air freshener could set off sneezing that turned into wheezing. Cleaning sprays, colognes, and the detergent aisle could all trigger it. Some nights, his heart pounded so hard he worried about a heart attack. He learned to recognize his house by its sounds: the bathroom fan, the fridge humming, anything to cover the sound of his heartbeat so he could sleep.

Doctors offered fragmented explanations: lingering COVID effects, anxiety, maybe mild asthma. He heard a lot of *probablys*. Inhalers gave minimal relief, and standard allergy medications barely touched the symptoms. James kept returning, insisting something deeper was wrong. He grew tired of being told to "give it time." Time was all he seemed to have, but none of it brought improvement.

The strain wasn't just physical—it was emotional, and it seeped into the corners of his life. His wife, practical and loving, was sympathetic at first, but as months dragged on without clear answers, impatience crept in. She wanted her husband back. Their kids didn't know what to do with a dad who used to organize impromptu backyard soccer and now sat out, watching from a lawn chair. His son teased him about being "out of shape," not realizing the sting behind the joke. His friends, not unkind but unseeing, rolled their eyes when he canceled plans yet again. They assumed he was exaggerating, that the shortness of breath and exhaustion couldn't be as bad as he claimed.

For James, that lack of belief cut deeper than the illness itself. He had built his identity on being capable and dependable. Now, not only was his body failing him, but the people closest to him thought he was being dramatic. There were nights he lay awake, staring at the ceiling, feeling both sick and utterly alone. He began to ration his words about symptoms to avoid the look—part pity, part doubt—that slipped across faces he loved.

Work complicated everything. The job sites he'd once navigated without a thought now felt like obstacle courses. Dust, paint fumes, solvents—what had always been background noise now triggered chest tightness and a metallic taste at the back of his throat. He found himself lingering outside buildings to let air circulate before stepping in. He planned site visits for cooler parts of the day to avoid the heat that intensified the breathlessness. On conference calls, he muted to cough, then unmuted with a cheerful tone he didn't feel. He learned to triage tasks: okay for the office, risky for the field, better delegated.

The crew noticed. They were loyal to him, but they also murmured. Was he okay? Was he up to it? That doubt echoed the doubt at home and bled into his own thinking.

What finally shifted the trajectory was a new specialist—an immunologist who listened without rushing him along. She didn't flinch at the crowded list of symptoms. She took in the wheeze and the racing heart, but also the flushing after meals, the headaches, the sudden collapse in heavily scented places. She explained mast cells in plain language—guard cells that can overreact after infections—and how that overreaction can look like a dozen different disorders stitched together. "We may be looking at Mast Cell Activation Syndrome," she said. The tests weren't tidy. Some lab results were normal. But the clinical pattern made sense. "We treat what's in front of us."

Treatment began with H1 and H2 antihistamines. Within a few weeks, his nightly wheezing softened. He still woke at times to that internal drumbeat, but the pounding after meals was less ferocious, and he slept a little easier. The improvement didn't feel like a miracle; it felt like someone had turned down the volume on the worst moments. That alone was enough to keep going.

A few weeks later, his doctor added montelukast, a leukotriene inhibitor taken at night, to target the stubborn, asthma-like piece of his symptoms. The change wasn't dramatic on day one, but it was unmistakable by week two. The tightness in his chest eased. The shortness of breath on the stairs began to calm. Those jolting, perfume-aisle wheeze attacks became fewer and further between. He noticed he was reaching for his rescue inhaler less often and waking up less congested. Dinners were interrupted less. Weekends included short drives without pulling over for a coughing fit. His doctor monitored him closely, checked in about side effects, and kept the regimen simple. With that oversight, montelukast became a steadying force, slotting neatly into the foundation built by the H1/H2 combination.

Even with progress, the emotional toll is carried forward. The family still didn't fully understand why he wasn't "better" yet. He looked almost normal—no oxygen tank, no cast or crutches—so the invisible weight was easy to underestimate. Frustrated, James began collecting articles from reputable medical journals and patient organizations about MCAS and long COVID. He printed them, highlighted the sections that mapped directly onto his life, and laid them out on the kitchen table one evening.

He didn't make a speech. He told the story plainly—what he felt, when it hit, what made it worse, and how the medications were helping. He showed them the science—that mast cells could misfire after viral infections, that this could cause heart and lung symptoms, that it wasn't in his head. He explained how perfumes, detergents, or even stress could tip his system over the edge, and he asked for specific changes: unscented laundry products, fragrance-free cleaners, and patience when a plan needed to shift. For once, instead of brushing him off, they listened. The evidence changed something. His wife's eyes softened in a way he hadn't seen in months. His son stopped joking and started offering to carry the heavy bags. His daughter asked, "What else can we do?" That night, James felt lighter—not because his symptoms vanished, but because he finally wasn't alone with them.

With his family on board, practical changes came quickly. They swapped detergents and fabric softeners. The glass cleaner and sprays were removed from the house, replaced by simple, fragrance-free alternatives. Windows were cracked open when the air felt heavy. A small air purifier hummed quietly in the living room. These adjustments didn't fix everything, but they meant the house stopped fighting him. Home became a place to recover, not an obstacle course to endure.

Work took longer. He set a meeting with his manager and laid out the situation without drama. He explained the triggers—fumes, solvents, strong fragrances—and proposed a plan: more office-based coordination, scheduling site visits for times with fewer exposures, and providing the option to step outside when needed. He wasn't asking to work less; he was asking to work smarter. To his surprise, the conversation went well. His manager wanted him functional rather than flattened. They adjusted his responsibilities so he could lead without constantly triggering symptoms. On site, he carried a small kit—antihistamines, inhaler, electrolyte tablets—and he gave himself permission to pause rather than push through. The crew saw that he still showed up, just differently. The whispering died down because the results spoke for themselves.

Alongside medication and environmental changes, James's immunologist suggested meditation—fifteen minutes a day, not to chase enlightenment but to give his nervous system a calmer set point. He had always dismissed meditation as something other people did. Sitting still with his thoughts sounded like a punishment, and the whole idea struck him as "hippie nonsense," a phrase he'd tossed around too easily. But the other tools were helping, and he realized the worst that could happen was that it did nothing. He tried.

The first sessions were clumsy. His legs twitched, his back ached, his mind wandered through to-do lists and stray worries. He hated it and kept going anyway—because stubbornness, when pointed in the right direction, is a tool. A few weeks in, he noticed something subtle. When a flare began—tight chest, quick breath—his mind didn't sprint quite as fast toward catastrophe. He could stay with the sensation long enough to see if it truly escalated, rather than pouring panic on top of it. The symptoms still came, but his reaction shifted. Meditation thinned the layer of fear that always made everything worse.

Daily life improved in small, concrete ways. Mornings weren't a coin toss. He learned which breakfasts didn't light a fuse (plain oats, eggs, rice), and he kept lunch predictable on workdays. He took short walks after dinner on the cooler streets, testing his edges without pushing them. Weekends were planned with back-up options: a café with outdoor seating, lawn bowls with the kids. The family adapted without resentment because they understood the why. That understanding turned friction into teamwork.

He also felt the change in his relationships. The kids began coming to him again—small things at first: "Can you look at my essay?" "Can you fix my bike brakes?" He realized how much he'd missed those ordinary requests. His wife noticed the difference, too. Late in the evening, they would sit together, and the conversation shifted from managing crises to sharing a day. There were still nights when his chest felt heavy and the cough returned, but they no longer defined the week.

None of this was linear. There were setbacks: a big deadline that meant late nights and a flare that followed; a friend's birthday in a crowded restaurant that loaded the air with cologne; a well-meaning visitor who wore strong perfume. But the bounce-back changed. A year earlier, a single exposure could have derailed him for a week. Now, with montelukast doing its quiet nightly work and the antihistamines steady in the background, the crash was shorter. Meditation helped him avoid feeding the fire with fear. If a shop was too busy, they would leave and laugh about it on the sidewalk, planning a different errand. Those small moments of choosing ease over stubbornness felt like wins in their own right.

He learned new boundaries at work, too. If a site suddenly reeked of fresh paint, he made the call: reschedule the interior walkthrough, handle logistics from outside, return when it was safe. He stopped pushing through in ways that only guaranteed he would pay later. That choice—less heroic in the moment, far wiser in the long run—kept him in the game.

A year after his diagnosis, James's life looked different, but it also looked solid. He still had MCAS, and long COVID had left its mark. He couldn't manage the fast group rides he loved, and crowded restaurants were still tricky. But he could breathe more easily, sleep more soundly, and walk around his neighborhood without counting steps or scouting for benches. He could sit through a full meal with his family without the sense that a starter pistol had gone off in his chest. He could plan a weekend that included something beyond recovery.

The base was H1 and H2 antihistamines. The turning point for his lungs was montelukast at night—unflashy, steady, the difference between a house that always smelled of smoke and one where the windows had finally been opened. The home changes mattered more than he'd guessed; living in air that didn't pick a fight with his body lowered the background noise. And the meditation gave him a way to meet a flare without making it bigger.

He's careful not to prescribe his path to anyone else. "Your body might respond differently," he says. "But the idea of a foundation holds: build what works, keep it steady, and don't light yourself on fire to keep up appearances." He remembers the day his family understood as the real turning point. "Not being believed was worse than being sick," he admits. "The day they got it, it was like my body exhaled. I wasn't fighting on two fronts anymore."

Now, progress isn't measured by grand gestures but by steady gains: fewer wheezing fits (especially after montelukast settled in), fewer terrifying heart palpitations, more days when he can sit with his family without feeling like a burden. He calls it good project management applied to health: set the plan, adjust when reality speaks, bank the wins, repeat. No miracles—just a life that works again.

James still has MCAS. He also has dinners that aren't cut short by breathlessness, weekend walks that end with conversation instead of panic, and a house that smells like... nothing at all. The big wins are made of small, repeated ones, and that, he's learned, is more than enough.

Michelle's Story:

Michelle was seventeen. It was her final year of high school, the year everyone told her she'd remember—the late-night study sessions, the lead-up to formal, the sense that life was about to break open and invite her in. Until the headaches started.

They weren't the kind that give up after a glass of water and a nap. They settled behind her eyes like a weight and set up camp. Her nose felt stuffed even when it wasn't, her sinuses throbbed as if she'd been swimming in a pool all day, and no amount of steam or saline washes seemed to help. She blamed hay fever at first, but winter changed nothing. She kept moving—school, netball, rehearsals for the end-of-year play—but there was a new drag in everything.

Around the same time, food got... strange. It started with meat—a burger that left her flushed and dizzy. Then yogurt. Then sauerkraut, which she'd been eating because someone on the internet said it was "good for the gut." Suddenly, the "healthy" foods were suspects. A week later, it was leftovers. Then a certain cheese. Then avocado. It felt like her body was drawing lines through her menus with a red pen. One afternoon, she ate a grilled chicken salad—the kind she'd had a hundred times—and found herself sitting in the bathroom stall at school, lightheaded and itchy, wondering what on earth was happening.

Michelle had grown up with a diagnosis of Ehlers–Danlos syndrome. Her joints were bendy; her skin bruised easily. She'd learned not to hyperextend her elbows and to tape her ankles for sport. Mostly, EDS had been something she lived alongside, not something that stopped her. She had a specialist she trusted—a calm, kind doctor who'd been with her family through growth spurts and sprains. When the headaches dug in and the weird food reactions piled up, she and her dad made an appointment.

They drove in during a full-blown flare. Her face was warm, her nose felt stuffed, and her head pounded. She felt miserable and, in a way, relieved—if something was going to show up on a test, this would be the moment. The doctor listened—really listened—and asked about timing, what she'd eaten, the perfumes in the school bathrooms, the cleaning sprays in the hallways. He nodded as a picture formed, then said he wanted to run labs right then, while her body was shouting. He mentioned mast cells in plain language—"sometimes these cells overreact; it can happen in people with EDS. We'll check."

They drew blood and sent urine samples. By the time she got home, she fell asleep on the couch with an ice pack on her face. A few days later, the results were back: her tryptase—one of the markers tied to mast cell activity—was abnormal during the flare, and a couple of other markers looked off, too. He called and didn't play games with uncertainty. He suspected Mast Cell Activation Syndrome. He said the term out loud and then translated it for a seventeen-year-old: "This is real. It has a name. And we can try things that help."

He started her on antihistamines. The plan was to take them regularly, not just "when it's bad," and keep track of symptoms. The first week didn't change her life, but it changed her days. The headaches eased, the sinus pressure lightened, allowing her to focus in class, and food reactions became less overwhelming. After school, she could lie down briefly and then actually get back up again.

But the disruption had already done its work. Teenagers organize life around small freedoms: grabbing sushi with friends after school, sharing chips at a movie, raiding the fridge at midnight. Michelle started saying no to invitations she would've leapt at last year. It wasn't just the food; it was the fear of feeling weird in front of everyone—the sudden flush, the itching, the dizzy spell that sent her to the bathroom. She kept a hoodie in her bag for scent-heavy classrooms and pulled up the hood when someone sprayed perfume in the row behind her. She learned where the quiet benches were on campus. She kept a small stash of safe snacks in her locker and backpack. Her friends were kind, but they didn't always get it. "Just take a Panadol," someone said once. She laughed to be polite and then went home to cry.

Her dad helped her reorganize the kitchen without making a big deal of it. They started freezing single portions to avoid the reactions to leftovers. They bought smaller amounts of fresh food and cooked more often. Michelle stopped pretending certain foods were fine just because she missed them. She let herself grieve pizza Fridays and then moved on. On the good days, she told herself that this was a season, not a sentence.

A month into antihistamines, Michelle went back to her doctor. He was pleased the edges were softening, but wanted to see if they could get her more stable. He suggested adding supplements and a couple of gentle herbal options that had been useful for other patients—nothing extreme, nothing meant to "fix" her overnight. The goal was simple: tamp down the overreactivity enough that her body had room to calm itself. She left with a plan: vitamin C in divided doses during the day, quercetin with meals, magnesium at night for nervous system steadiness, and a turmeric/curcumin blend introduced in small amounts. He taught her the trick of starting low, going slow, and changing one thing at a time so she could see what actually helped.

The sinus pain shifted from relentless to occasional. The daily headache turned into a few times a week, then once a week, then only around her period or after a truly stressful day. Her brain felt clearer. In class, she could follow a complicated discussion and remember what she wanted to say without panic. The foods she tolerated expanded—not back to "everything," but enough to make school lunches and social life easier. Chicken and rice gave way to fresh fish, certain fruits, and a few vegetables that were once considered risky. She learned that some foods were fine if they were cooked and eaten immediately, but trouble if they sat in the fridge. Taking vitamin C consistently mattered more than she'd expected, and magnesium at night meant fewer mornings where she woke up already depleted.

The ripple effects were real. Studying stopped feeling like trying to read through a smear on the page. She could sit for longer without her neck and face throbbing. She started doing homework at the library again, where the air felt clean and quiet. Her marks steadied. Getting that back—being able to concentrate, to contribute, to feel like yourself in class—felt like someone had opened a window.

Her friends adjusted with her. They planned picnics where everyone brought their own food. They found a café with outdoor seating that would cook simple meals the way Michelle needed. "Does this work for you?" became normal. As for the school formal, Michelle decided she wanted to go. She did what she did best now: planned. She ate safe foods during the day, packed an emergency kit (antihistamines, electrolytes, a protein bar she trusted), and made a plan to step outside if the room got too scented. She still danced. She still laughed with her friends. She still cried a little on the drive home—tired, yes, but also relieved that she hadn't had to sit on the sidelines of her own life.

Not every day was easy. There were weeks when stress stacked up—exams, rehearsals, the messy parts of friendship—and her symptoms hummed louder. Sometimes the weather made her sinuses heavy again. Sometimes a teacher sprayed air freshener, and the whole room felt tilted. But now she had levers to pull: adjust supplements, focus on fresh foods, hydrate, and rest earlier. The symptoms that used to spiral felt more like waves—still real, but less likely to knock her flat.

The best part was feeling seen. Her doctor never made her feel like she was exaggerating. He reminded her and her dad that quick testing during flares had given them useful clues—like the abnormal tryptase—and that her response to treatment mattered as much as labs. He told her to trust her own observations. That permission was medicine in its own way. It meant she didn't have to spend energy proving her experience to anyone.

Michelle became quietly skilled at advocating for herself. She spoke with the school office about keeping her classroom as fragrance-free as possible, and to their credit, they tried. She emailed teachers before big events to ask for a seat near an open window. She learned to say, "I can't do that, but I can do this," and to offer alternatives rather than apologize. Most people wanted to help; they just needed to know how.

At home, she reclaimed the parts of life that make being seventeen fun. She made a playlist for car rides to school with her younger brother. She FaceTimed her best friend while they studied—cameras on, mics off, just company. Saturday morning, waffles came back—now a simple recipe with ingredients that didn't set her off, hot from the pan and eaten right away. She and her dad started a ritual of cooking double and freezing half, not just to protect against leftovers but to save future Michelle from a bad day. Small systems, big relief.

There were also new habits that didn't feel like chores. On Sundays, she set out her supplements in a little organizer so she didn't have to think about them during the week. She kept a soft eye mask and a water bottle on her nightstand. She took five minutes after school to sit on the back steps and breathe before diving into homework. These weren't punishments; they were kindnesses—ways to give her body a head start.

Slowly, life stopped being about what she'd lost and started being about what she'd redesigned. She still had EDS. She still had a sensitive system that liked fresh food and simple routines. She still had to say no to certain things. But she also had friends who'd meet her in the park instead of the food court, a family that kept the house low-scent and calm, and a doctor who treated her as a partner. The combination—antihistamines, a thoughtful supplement and herbal plan, practical food strategies, and steady support—let her be a student again, a friend again, a teenager again.

The school year ticked forward. Her headaches were no longer the headline. Sinus days still happened, but they didn't take over the week. The food list stopped growing and, little by little, began to loosen. She learned what worked for her body and what didn't, and she stopped apologizing for honoring that. When teachers handed out end-of-year awards, Michelle didn't expect anything. But in her English class, the teacher called her name for a quiet recognition—resilience, yes, but also contribution. "For showing up—really showing up," the teacher said, smiling. Heat rose in her face, but it wasn't a flare. It was pride.

If you asked her what changed the most, she wouldn't say "everything." She'd say, "Enough." Enough relief from the antihistamines that her days were no longer narrowed to that pain behind her eyes. Enough calm from the supplements and herbs that her body didn't ping-pong from food reaction to food reaction. She had enough support at home and at school that she could stop bracing and start living. She still carries a little kit in her backpack. She still reads labels. She still leaves a room if it's too scented. Now those choices feel like taking care of herself, not missing out.

On the night the results came out for university entrance, she and her friends gathered at a friend's house. There was a table with plain rice, grilled fish, and fruit—simple, safe, delicious. They laughed, screamed, and took photos in the backyard fairy lights. Michelle's phone buzzed. She opened the link and saw her number. It was enough to get into the program she'd hoped for. Her dad hugged her; her brother shouted; her friends jumped up and down. For a second, Michelle let herself rewind the tape—bathroom stalls and thudding heartbeats, red pens through menus, afternoons where the headache made the world small—and then she pressed play on what was right in front of her.

Life became possible in all the best ways. She planned her next steps with the same practical care she'd learned this year: find housing with a decent kitchen, keep a low-scent roommate agreement, register with campus disability services in case she needed quiet exam rooms or flexible attendance during flares, locate the nearby farmers' market so she could keep cooking fresh. She wasn't scared of university. She was ready, in the way that comes from having already solved harder problems than most people could see.

When people asked how she was doing now, Michelle didn't give a medical lecture. She said, "Better. Really better." Then, if they wanted more, she'd add, "My doctor saw me on a bad day, ran tests that actually caught what was going on, and started me on antihistamines. Supplements and a couple of gentle herbs made a big difference. I keep food simple and fresh. My family and school helped. It's not perfect, but it's good. I'm good."

There's a photo from that night—Michelle in a simple dress, hair swept back, smiling with her whole face. If you look closely, you can see a small crossbody bag at her side. Inside are the things she carries now without shame: antihistamines, a safe snack, a tiny bottle of electrolytes. Tools, not fears. Prepared, not panicked. A seventeen-year-old who had a year stolen and then, with help, patience, and a steady plan, took it back.

Aaron's Story:

The hiss of the kettle filled the quiet room, marking the start of another carefully measured day. Aaron, at twenty-nine, kept things simple: laptop open, two solid hours of work, then a pause. He rented a ground-floor apartment, a desk by the window, and used a straightforward weekly calendar to keep his days steady and bite-sized. For twelve years, almost half his life, POTS and ME/CFS had trimmed his routine down to what he could reliably manage. He kept things orderly because it kept him going: compression socks folded on the chair arm, electrolytes lined up on the counter, a short list of meals his body tolerated, a doctor who knew his history, and a handful of online friends who understood the long, quiet stretches. It wasn't the life he'd imagined, but it was the one he could sustain—steady, pared back, and built around energy he had to spend like a scarce currency.

He was meticulous because he had to be. Mornings started slowly. He moved like a diver surfacing—careful, measured, listening for warning signs. Before he stood, he salted a glass of water and drank it in slow swallows. Sometimes he leaned against the wall on the way to the kitchen, because the world tilted without asking. Showering was a strategy: lukewarm, quick, a stool, door slightly open. Breakfast was always the same—something bland, something he knew wouldn't send his heart galloping. Then two hours of work followed by rest, because that was what kept the day from collapsing.

People drifted in and out of view like passing trains. He ordered groceries on his phone. He texted his mother every evening, short and cheerful, because she worried less if he sounded fine. When friends invited him to birthdays or barbecues, he sent gifts and excuses. It wasn't that he didn't want to go; it was that his body couldn't be trusted. A crowded room meant perfumes, heat, laughter rising and falling like waves he couldn't ride. A late night meant a crash that might last a week. And not knowing when the crash would come—that was the part that kept him cautious and home.

His doctor—steady, kind, careful—had been with him since the beginning. They had built a plan that kept Aaron afloat: fluids, salt, compression, pacing, and a list of medications to ease the worst of the dizziness and headaches. It wasn't a cure, not even close, but it was a raft. And when you're adrift for a decade, a raft is something.

The push to try something different didn't come from a clinic or a paper. It came from an online friend named Theo, a person Aaron had never met in real life but who somehow knew how to ask the right questions. They messaged back and forth most nights: symptoms, experiments, the small workarounds that make a day livable. One evening, after Aaron described how crowded stores and leftover food were setting him off—flushing, itching, brain fog slamming down like a shutter—Theo wrote, "Have you ever looked into mast cells? MCAS?" The letters felt like a foreign country. Aaron filed them away with skepticism. He already had a diagnosis; he didn't need another.

But the idea wouldn't leave him alone. He started noticing patterns he had glossed over. The way a hot apartment and a stressful email could team up to steal his afternoon. The way certain foods lit a fuse. The way a neighbor's laundry detergent seeped under his door and made his heart tap faster. He saw how these moments weren't random; they were a language he hadn't learned to read.

Theo nudged again: "Maybe get a second opinion? Someone who knows MCAS." It felt like a betrayal to consider, because Aaron's doctor had been good to him all these years. But good doctors can miss things when a body is complicated. He asked for a referral anyway.

The new physician—an internal medicine doctor with a focus on autonomic disorders—didn't promise miracles. She did something better: she asked for a full story and listened without interrupting. She didn't flinch when

Aaron recited the catalogue—dizziness when standing, racing heart for no clear reason, headaches behind his eyes, bone-deep fatigue, rashes that came and went, episodes of weird flushing after meals, a fog so thick he could lose his own train of thought mid-sentence. She asked when the worst reactions happened, what he was doing, what he'd eaten, and what the room smelled like. When he finished, she said, "ME/CFS and POTS explain a lot. But you may also have mast cell activation in the mix. It would fit the way heat, stress, and certain foods tip you over."

She ordered tests. Nothing heroic—just the right labs at the right time, including a plan to draw blood during a flare rather than on a "good" morning when his body was quiet. On a day when his heart wouldn't stop hammering and his skin itched in waves, he went for the blood draw and dutifully collected the urine samples she'd requested. A few days later, her office called. Some markers looked off. Nothing alone was dramatic, but together—with his history and how he reacted to triggers—they made a case for mast cell activation sitting alongside his POTS and ME/CFS.

They began H1 and H2 antihistamines on a regular schedule. The flushing after meals eased a notch. That constant prickle under his skin—the one he'd mistaken for anxiety—quieted. He still had bad hours, but fewer avalanches. For the first time in years, he could make coffee without immediately sitting down afterward to wait out a storm of palpitations.

At the second visit, the doctor said gently, "I'd like to try something else—low dose naltrexone. It sometimes helps calm the immune system and can be useful in ME/CFS. It won't fix everything, but it may turn the volume down." She explained what to watch for: sleep disruption at first, vivid dreams, a kind of jangly adjustment.

He took the first small dose on a Tuesday night, placed the pill on his tongue like a small dare, and went to bed. His hand almost trembled as he lifted the water glass, a mix of dread and hope coiling in his stomach. The change arrived quickly, unpleasant and promising all at once. He slept badly, tossing and dreaming in bright colors that clung to him like static when he opened his eyes. But quietly, strangely, his body felt calmer. The morning didn't greet him with the usual electric hum under his skin. His heart still sped up when he stood, but the surge was less spiky, less panicked. He noticed he could read a short article all the way through without his brain skipping like a scratched CD. It wasn't comfort, not yet, but it was a shift.

The second night was worse. He lay awake and watched the ceiling shadows move as cars passed outside. By morning, he was irritated with himself for hoping. "Of course it's not going to work," he muttered, and made toast he didn't want. But he kept going because he'd promised to try for two weeks unless something truly awful happened. Through those first ten days, sleep was a mess, and daytime carried a new steadiness. By the end of week two, the awful dreams dulled down, and his body kept settling. He emailed the doctor: "Sleep bad, symptoms... muted?" It wasn't scientific language, but it was accurate.

In the third week, the change moved from interesting to undeniable. He woke one morning and realized he didn't feel like he was made of glass. He stood up slowly, as always, but this time the room didn't swing quite so hard. He walked to the kitchen, poured water, and didn't need to lean on the counter. It was ordinary and astonishing. He messaged Theo: "LDN is doing... something."

Progress didn't arrive in a straight line. There were jagged days that reminded him of the old pattern—heatwave afternoons when his pulse raced for no reason, anxious mornings when sleep debt made everything louder. But even on those days, the floor sat higher. He didn't slam into it as easily. The antihistamines did their steady background work; the low dose naltrexone seemed to coax his system out of constant alarm.

He began testing small changes, the way you do when trust creeps back into your bones. He tried a five-minute walk on a quiet street at noon instead of at dusk when it was cooler. He took his laptop to the kitchen table instead of working from bed, and lasted an extra half hour before his body asked for rest. He washed a sinkful of dishes in one go. It sounds like nothing until you remember the years that trained him to break every task into five parts to avoid crashing.

By the second month on the new regimen, sleep had transformed from terrible to deep. He woke before his alarm—something that hadn't happened in years—and lay there noticing the quiet in his body, like a street at 5 a.m. before the city wakes. Sometimes his dreams were still vivid, but they no longer left him wrung out. He began to trust bedtime again.

Energy behaved differently too. With ME/CFS, exertion had always carried a delayed cost he couldn't predict. Now the cost was smaller, more negotiable. If he watered the plants and answered emails and cooked a meal, he didn't automatically lose the next day. If he did too much and started to tip, he could often pull back in time and recover by evening. It was a new kind of math—still careful, still humble, but not governed entirely by fear.

His house changed with him. The blinds went up during the day, letting in light he used to block because brightness seemed to hijack his nervous system. He bought a small table fan, not to battle sweats but to make the space feel breezy and awake. He reorganized his pantry around foods he trusted—fresh meats cooked and frozen in single portions, rice, eggs, and simple vegetables. He stopped punishing himself for not being "adventurous" with food and instead celebrated the meals that left his body calm.

With calm came appetite for connection—a strange, tender hunger. He started saying yes to daytime things. A friend offered to meet for a ten-minute walk at the quiet end of the park. Another friend asked if he could help choose a secondhand desk; they met at a thrift store mid-morning on a Tuesday when the aisles were empty. He drove there himself and sat in the car afterward with his hands on the steering wheel, smiling at nothing.

The loneliness that had settled in him over the years didn't vanish; it thawed. He realized how much of his personality had been in storage—humor kept private, opinions saved for message boards because typing didn't trigger a crash the way talking did. In person, he heard himself make a joke and saw someone laugh. It startled him in a good way.

He joined a small, local group that met outdoors twice a month, where people read poetry or shared short stories. He didn't read; he just listened, a folding chair in the shade, electrolyte water in a bottle by his foot. One woman wore a floral perfume that might have bothered him before, but the breeze and his steadier body made it tolerable. He drove home with the windows down.

Work changed too. He increased his daily "focus window" by fifteen minutes at a time, watching carefully for that familiar crash feeling. He set a timer and rested before his nerves demanded it. A funny thing happened—productive hours expanded when he "spent" them more gently. He added small video calls he used to avoid because screen time seemed to drain him. Seeing faces lifted something he hadn't realized was heavy. His manager noticed the difference in his availability, but more importantly, in his mood. He said as much in a quarterly check-in. "You sound... lighter," he offered. Aaron said, "I feel... steadier." It was the best word he had.

None of this erased twelve years of hard living. He still had POTS. He still managed ME/CFS like a careful accountant, counting spoons. Heat waves could still knock him down. Loud, crowded spaces were still risky. But the texture of his days changed, from survival to something that included choice. And choice is a kind of joy.

He kept seeing both doctors—the longtime physician who knew his history and the new one who understood mast cells. There was no drama in that; it turned out to be the best of both worlds. They compared notes when needed. They changed nothing quickly. They added nothing fancy. The heart of the plan stayed simple: H1 and H2 antihistamines on schedule, low dose naltrexone slowly titrated, hydration and salt for POTS, compression when standing in lines or cooking, fresh food routines, early bedtimes more nights than not. He kept a small emergency kit in his glove compartment and another by the door: antihistamines, electrolytes, and a simple snack. Preparedness made it easier to say yes.

One afternoon, months into this new phase, he found himself at a café at 10:30 a.m.—an hour that used to be dangerous because mornings were often the most fragile. He sat at an outdoor table with a friend and ordered tea. He ate a slice of plain toast because he still played it safe. He laughed. He watched people pass with dogs, prams, and grocery bags. When he stood to leave, the world didn't tilt. He didn't need to stare at the horizon and breathe through a surge of adrenaline. He just stood. On the drive home, he took the longer route because the light through the trees was incredible, and he suddenly remembered that life can be beautiful at 10:58 a.m. on a weekday.

He made two new friendships that stuck, the kind you build on the ground you have, not the ground you wish you had. They were daytime friends, walking friends, quiet-errand friends. He didn't perform wellness for them. On bad days, he texted, "Rain check?" and they said, "Of course." On good days, they met for an hour and then everyone went home happy.

He also did a brave, ordinary thing: he told his mother the truth about the changes without promising a future he couldn't guarantee. "I'm doing better," he said on a Sunday call. "I don't know how far this goes, but I'm driving again during the day, and the medicine is helping me feel steadier." She cried, not with worry but with the kind of relief that sneaks up on you after years of holding your breath.

There were stumbles. An enthusiastic attempt at tidying the whole apartment in one go landed him in bed for the afternoon with warning signs—buzzing heart, cotton-wool brain. He didn't spiral into self-blame. He adjusted, learned, and kept the gains. A loud afternoon in a hardware store reminded him that fluorescent lights and chemical aisles were still not his friends; he left, sat in the car, and laughed at himself for thinking he could do everything at once just because he felt better. Progress is a conversation, not a lecture. He was learning to listen.

Around nine months after he started the new regimen, a friend asked him what he wanted to do with a Saturday. He didn't know how to answer at first because Saturdays used to be for recovery. He said, "Maybe we can drive to the lake. Sit on a bench. You can fish if you want. I'll read." They went. He packed water and snacks, wore a hat, and looked for shade as second nature. He didn't swim. He didn't hike. He sat, read, and watched the light move across the water. He sent a photo to Theo—the friend who'd started this particular domino run—with the caption: "Out. In the daytime. On purpose." Theo replied with a string of celebratory emojis and a message that said simply, "Knew you had it in you."

Life is not a montage of victories. It is a series of days. But when the texture of those days lifts from grey to colored, you notice. Aaron noticed. He began to look ahead in small ways: renew his driver's license without anxiety, say yes to a mid-morning haircut, water his plants every Tuesday so he'd remember that time was passing and he was living in it.

If you asked him to sum up the change, he would choose his words carefully. "I'm not cured. I also don't live in the same body I did a year ago. The mast cell meds helped. Low dose naltrexone helped in a way I could feel—sleep first, then everything else. I still manage POTS and ME/CFS every day. But the volume is lower. I can go out in the daytime. I can drive. I can have an hour with a friend and come home with energy left. That's... good. That's life."

And then he would probably offer you a glass of salted water, out of habit and kindness, because those two things are how he learned to live again.

Nina's Story:

Nina felt it first, like an electric charge touching her lips, then a tightening in her throat, as if a drawstring were pulling closed. She was at a café, a familiar spot with the usual chatter from the barista and the cool air from the door mixing with the scent of freshly brewed coffee. It was a salad she'd ordered before. Her heart kicked into an off-beat sprint, and her knees trembled. By the time her partner Marc got her to the emergency room, each breath felt like pulling air through a narrow straw.

The doctors eased the immediate danger, but not the lingering fear that her body could turn on her without warning. After that day, every meal became a question mark.

Nina was thirty-four, a graphic designer in a small coastal city where mornings smelled like salt and coffee. Her days looked neat from the outside: clean layouts, loyal clients, a partner she adored, friends who texted her memes before she'd finished her first cup. She hit deadlines, sent thank-you notes, and remembered birthdays. The version of Nina most people met was capable and bright. What they didn't see was the shadow that moved with her everywhere: the constant risk of anaphylaxis. It wasn't dramatic most days. It was quieter than that, a hum under every choice, a calculation before every bite, a scan of every room for what might be invisible and dangerous.

She stopped eating out almost entirely. Her kitchen became a refuge and command center. Cutting boards were bleached before and after use. Utensils were color-coded, and jars labeled with purchase dates in tidy handwriting. If a spice blend didn't list every ingredient, it stayed on the shelf. Leftovers older than a day went straight to the bin. She began to notice a new pattern—perfumes, detergents, and cleaning products could set her off fast. She switched to fragrance-free basics and drew a clear boundary between her space and others'. Cross-contamination was no longer theoretical. Safety lived in the details.

Preparedness wasn't a phase; it became a practice. She kept epinephrine everywhere—one in her bag, one in Marc's car, a third in her desk drawer. She checked expiration dates as regularly as she watered the plants. A coworker joked once about her "portable pharmacy," and Nina didn't laugh. For her, being ready wasn't paranoia. It was how she kept herself alive.

The scariest part wasn't only the anaphylaxis. It was the way fear seeped into ordinary tasks until everything felt like it might be a test she could fail. Grocery shopping turned into reconnaissance: scanning labels, looking for hidden oils and vague "natural flavors," putting things back because the risk of ambiguity was too high. Invitations required choreography: No fragrances, please; no new cleaning products; no food prepared in the same space as shellfish. People tried to be kind. Most were. But even kindness sometimes carried a flicker of confusion in the eyes of the person across from her, the smallest question mark that made her feel like she was asking too much, or making it up, or both. Isolation doesn't arrive like a storm; it spreads like fog. She found herself saying no more often than she wanted to, building weekends that were safe and, too often, lonely.

Doctors made the fog thicker before it thinned. Allergy panels came back inconclusive. A clinician suggested stress. Another wondered, gently, if she might be "overly vigilant." The language was careful. The effect wasn't. Each appointment that ended with a shrug made her doubt herself in new ways. If the salad that nearly closed her airway didn't leave a clear fingerprint in her labs, what did that mean? Was she failing to describe it correctly? Was she losing her mind? She cut herself into smaller shapes—maybe if she were less precise, she'd be believed; maybe if she were more precise. None of it worked. The body keeps its own counsel.

The turning point came with a doctor who properly listened. He didn't watch the clock when she described the café. He didn't flinch at the mismatch between one week's reaction and the next week's non-reaction to the same food. He talked about mast cells—immune sentinels found almost everywhere in the body that, in some people, become over-responsive—and how they can release surges of chemical messengers unpredictably, sometimes without a single clear allergen to blame. He said the words she needed, plainly: *Mast Cell Activation Syndrome*. It wasn't a finish line. It was a map.

A diagnosis didn't shrink the risk, but it changed the story she told herself about it. She wasn't imagining things. She wasn't fragile. She was living with a condition that medicine was still learning how to name, measure, and treat. Her treatment began with H1 and H2 antihistamines. Hives arrived with less violence. Flushing cooled faster. The hair-trigger feeling backed off half a step.

Her doctor added sodium cromolyn before meals, explaining it simply. "It helps mast cells keep their messengers in their pockets," he said. The first week brought a new discomfort—bloating that made her want to quit. He had warned her this might happen. She stuck it out. By the third week, the change surprised her. Reactions that used to hit like tidal waves turned into choppy seas that she could ride out. Her stomach wasn't a battlefield every day. She could eat small, fresh meals without bracing for impact. She started freezing portions the same day she cooked them and felt like she'd wrestled back a piece of ordinary life she thought she'd lost.

Her doctor encouraged her to create an emergency plan of practical steps to steady her nerves. Not as a jinx, but to lower the temperature of fear. Nina wrote step-by-step instructions: what to do, when to use the EpiPen, when to call, and when to go. She kept a copy in her bag, on the fridge, and at work. She handed one to Marc and watched his face as he read it. "We're going to be okay," he said. "And I'm grateful to know exactly what to do." Giving the plan to her manager felt like making a fuss. She slid it across the desk anyway. Her manager read it, nodded, and said, "Thank you. I'm glad to have this." A coworker told her, "I'd want us to be prepared." The awkwardness eased. Readiness became a way to bring people closer, not push them away.

Nina didn't attempt a grand return to "normal." She chose gentle re-entry. Picnics instead of restaurants, where she could bring her own food and write her own rules. Coffee outdoors, where the air circulated and the fragrance from someone's shampoo didn't pool around her. Short walks along the water during off-hours. She left early when she needed to. It wasn't heroic; it was deliberate. Confidence didn't fall from the sky. It grew in increments.

Even as routines steadied, the horizon still held storms. There were quiet weeks. There were sudden, baffling reactions. After one rough month with two episodes that accelerated quickly, her immunologist raised the possibility of trying Xolair (omalizumab), a biologic that targets IgE, the antibody involved in allergic reactions. It wasn't a guarantee, he said, and it wasn't right for everyone. But some people with severe, allergic-type MCAS flares found the edge less sharp on it. Hope is a complicated thing when you've had to ration it. Nina didn't leap; she asked questions. Risks, benefits, and monitoring. What would it change about her day? What would it not change at all?

They started cautiously. The first injections set, with a nurse following up after each one. Nina left the rest untouched: antihistamines, pre-meal cromolyn, her emergency kit, and the plan she carried. A month passed without a headline. Somewhere in the second, the weather shifted inside her body so quietly she almost missed it. A meal that might have left her flushing and dizzy... didn't. A whiff of perfume in a shop sent her toward the door, but her throat stayed open. She realized one afternoon that she hadn't used her EpiPen in weeks. The fear that usually sat like a weight on her chest when she ate anywhere but home lightened a notch. She still respected labels and limits. She still mapped exits. But the constant red alert softened.

By the third month, coincidence didn't feel like a good enough explanation. The reactions that used to sprint toward anaphylaxis stalled earlier, like a match that fizzled instead of catching. She hadn't needed epinephrine once in that stretch. She said yes to a friend's backyard barbecue and took her own food, setting boundaries, but actually going. She sat through a long afternoon meeting without rehearsing the emergency steps in her head. She fell asleep without replaying the first awful event in the cafe. The changes didn't arrive with trumpets. They arrived in the small spaces where fear had lived and now, suddenly, didn't.

Work looked different when fear took up less room. She could focus through the 3 p.m. drag that used to set off a fog of vigilance. She asked for unscented office supplies and a fragrance-free bubble around her desk. Because she was present more consistently, the requests landed as reasonable rather than dramatic. Her manager noticed the way she now sat in a room: less on guard, more herself.

Nina is careful not to tell the story like a miracle. Xolair didn't make her fearless. It made her feel safe enough to live. The difference matters. She kept up regular check-ins with her doctor, the foundation of antihistamines and cromolyn, the emergency plan, and the kit in her bag. She counted every win: a meal eaten without panic, a morning that didn't start with dread, an afternoon that didn't require a nap to shut down a reaction that almost happened. Setbacks came—they still do. A new scented cleaner at a friend's house sent her to sit in the car with the windows down. A mystery seasoning at a restaurant she tried to rejoin gave her a rough night. But rough nights didn't spiral into emergencies as often. The floor of her health rose. Experiments no longer felt like a dare; they felt like practice.

There was one more piece that surprised her. Nina had spent months unlearning the idea that her symptoms were "in her head." She wasn't eager to pick up anything that sounded like it might suggest otherwise. Still, in late evenings when fear felt sticky, she found herself reading about nervous-system work—brain retraining programs that didn't deny biology so much as coach the body out of threat mode. People described short practices, used consistently, that softened the reflexive alarm that made everything worse. She didn't want magical thinking. She wanted something grounded enough to try without hating herself for trying.

She chose a program that was quiet rather than flashy. Five to ten minutes, several times a day, not a life overhaul. She practiced in small loops: notice the room; let her eyes land on something neutral or kind (the bend of light along the counter, the sound of the kettle); say honest words out loud—"safe enough right now"; let her shoulders drop an inch; return to what she was doing. She took the practice outside the house in tiny tests she could control—

walk past the laundry aisle at the supermarket, step outside, breathe, reset. A perfumed elevator had once flipped a switch in her whole body. Now, she could feel the first edge of heat, step out on the next floor, and interrupt the story that used to run ahead of her. The body still reacted sometimes. The mind stopped piling fear onto it quite so fast.

The nervous system work made room for the medications to do their job. The medications made it easier to practice calmly. Cromolyn kept meals from feeling like roulette. Antihistamines lowered the hum. Xolair pulled her back from the cliff edge so a spark didn't find kindling every time. The emergency plan lowered the temperature of worst-case scenarios. The kit in her bag replaced superstition with steps. It wasn't just one single thing.

Nina began saying yes more often. A small concert. A seat on the aisle, exits noted, emergency kit packed, safe dinner eaten first. Fear hummed under her ribs—she didn't pretend it didn't—but it didn't drown her out. When the music started, she let herself lean into it. She stood. She swayed. She laughed under string lights with Marc, and for once, the night was about the song and not survival. On the way home she cried, the kind of quiet tears that have less to do with the event and more to do with the fact that a moment can be just a moment again.

She told a few more people, carefully, about her plan. A neighbor who liked to chat in the hallway agreed to keep the floor unscented on days when Nina needed the elevator. A friend lit candles only after Nina left. Small accommodations didn't feel like special treatment anymore; they felt like community.

At work, she started training a junior designer and was surprised by how much she enjoyed it. She would have said no to that kind of responsibility a year ago. Now, mentoring felt right; with a run of steady days, she could rely on the month ahead. She still blocked out a few short breaks in her calendar each day. No one needed to know those five minutes were for nervous-system practice, not emails. She wrote "reset" in her planner and followed through with it.

Not every morning is easy. Some days still arrive with a tremor. She has had stretches where a rash blooms and fades for no reason she can name. She left a movie twenty minutes in because someone arrived wearing a cloud of fragrance, and the room wasn't ventilated enough to make it bearable. Leaving is part of the plan, too. That's what preparedness gives you—permission to change your mind without calling it failure.

She keeps a small sketch of her local coastline on the fridge. The lighthouse, jetty, and tide pools with "Possible" written underneath, because those are places she never expected to go again, but now she can. Some spots are still off-limits, yet more feel possible, and the path between them is clearer; even sitting on the porch after dinner counts as real progress.

She isn't fearless, but she's prepared—epinephrine at hand, clear boundaries around exposures, steady follow-up care—and she now measures a good life by its steadiness and the space it leaves for laughter.

There are mornings when she wakes and feels the old habit of dread reach for her. This is when the steps she's practiced do their quiet work. She orients. She says the line she wrote for herself: "safe enough right now". She gets out of bed, opens the window, and lets the sea and the coffee smell in. She feeds the cat. She texts her friend back. She makes a list that is short, honest, and doable. She forgets to be brave, and is anyway.

If you asked her what changed, she could tell it as a sequence. MCAS gave her a name. Antihistamines lowered the hum. Cromolyn turned meals from tidal waves to choppy seas. A written plan made preparedness shareable. Xolair dulled the edge of the worst reactions. Nervous-system practice made her less likely to pour gasoline on sparks. But she might also just say: I kept adding small things until the day arrived where I felt like I had found a place I could stay.

Nina still lives with MCAS. She respects the landscape, but the map is different now. The tempo of her life is quieter; there's room for work, friendship, and ordinary joy, not just survival. On her desk is a tiny sticker she made for herself: progress, not performance. It is not inspirational. It is precise. It is how she walks through her days.

Conclusion

Your Path Forward

You've travelled a long road through these pages. You've explored what mast cell activation syndrome is, how it can touch so many parts of life, and the many ways people approach care—from conventional medicine to natural therapies, from lifestyle shifts to building a personal plan. If you've come this far, you've gathered more than just information. You've gathered perspective, language, and maybe even a sense of connection to something bigger than your own experience.

This book hasn't promised a magic cure or a straight-line path, because life with MCAS rarely follows those rules. What it has offered is something perhaps more valuable: a set of tools, a collection of stories, and a way of seeing your journey that centers not just on survival, but on living well—on reclaiming moments of joy, connection, and purpose even in the face of uncertainty.

So as these pages come to a close, take a moment to reflect on the ground already covered and consider how the insights gained here can shape the next steps in your journey. Ask yourself, "What can I try this week?" By identifying a single, actionable step, you can begin translating your reflections into meaningful action.

Looking Back on the Road Travelled

When MCAS first came into view, it may have brought both relief and overwhelm—finally a name for what was happening, but also a new layer of complexity. Learning the basics of mast cells and their role in widespread symptoms helped turn confusion into clarity.

Early on, the medical language felt foreign: tryptase, histamine, stabilizers. Over time, those terms connected the dots, showing why one trigger could spark reactions that looked like allergies, asthma, and anxiety all at once. For many, this recognition brought validation after years of dismissal.

Diagnosis carried mixed emotions—relief that the condition is real, frustration with inconsistent testing, and empowerment in learning how to advocate for care. Treatment unfolded as both science and art: medications, supplements, and lifestyle strategies woven together differently for each person. Food, stress management, and nervous system support proved just as central as prescriptions.

Adjusting the environment—choosing safer products, protecting sleep, filtering air—became another form of medicine. What once felt like a burden began to look more like creating breathing space.

Finally, the journey became about taking action: building a care team, teaching loved ones, tracking your progress, and adjusting as time goes on. These chapters are not a map, but more like a compass, pointing you toward balance, resilience, and the confidence to keep moving forward.

Letting Go of Perfection

One of the most important threads woven through this book is the reminder that "living well" with MCAS does not mean being symptom-free, perfectly disciplined, or endlessly strong. Living well means building a life where your condition is part of the picture, but not the whole canvas. In this journey, you might ask yourself, "What if I let others see my struggle?" Embracing vulnerability can be daunting, but it allows for deeper connections and understanding. Consider the story of a reader who, instead of hiding her challenges, shared them with her community, finding grace and acceptance not in perfection, but in the courage to be authentic. This act of imperfect courage illuminated her path, showing that embracing one's full truth can also lead to self-compassion and growth.

Think of life as a garden. MCAS might be a large bed in your garden, maybe even one that dominates the center. But around it, you can plant seeds and tend areas of joy, love, creativity, friendship, rest, and purpose. Those plantings don't erase the MCAS bed, but they keep it from being the only thing you see.

For some people, the temptation is to turn management into a rigid checklist. Every food logged, every supplement timed, every flare scrutinized. While structure can help, it can also become its own kind of prison. This is where self-compassion matters most. It is not about "doing everything right"—it is about creating space for flexibility, rest, and even mistakes.

There will be setbacks. There will be flares that blindside you even when you've done "everything right." There will be days when the best you can do is breathe, hydrate, and ride out the discomfort. That does not mean you're failing. It means you're human, living with a condition that is unpredictable by nature.

Rather than aiming for perfection, try to notice what patterns help you. What usually makes things easier? What helps you enjoy the things that matter most? Healing is often less about getting rid of every symptom and more about slowly making life feel better, step by step.

Perfection is not the goal. Compassion—for yourself, for your system, for your process—is.

Truths to Carry WIth You

So how do you take the threads of this book and weave them into your daily life? Here are some truths that may help anchor you:

- **You are the expert of your own body.** Doctors, researchers, and books can provide knowledge and options, but only you can feel what is happening inside you. Trust that wisdom.

- **Small changes matter.** A single adjustment—whether it's removing one trigger food, adding one supportive supplement, or creating one calming bedtime ritual—can shift your baseline more than you expect. Healing often happens through accumulation, not overnight transformation.
- **Flexibility is your ally.** Your needs will change. What helps today may not help tomorrow. That's not failure—that's part of the process. Staying open, curious, and adaptable will serve you far more than rigid rules.
- **Community is medicine.** Support groups, advocacy networks, and friendships with people who "get it" are not optional extras. They are as vital as any pill or supplement. Isolation weakens us; connection strengthens us.
- **Joy is not frivolous—it's essential.** Pursuing joy does not mean ignoring illness. It means refusing to let illness have the final word. A laugh with a friend, a walk under the trees, a hobby that lights you up—these are not distractions. They are lifelines.

Emotional Well-Being: A Gentle Note

If you take nothing else from these pages, let it be this: You are not broken. You are not "too much." You are not alone.

MCAS is complicated, but it does not erase your worth or your potential. You have already proven your resilience by reading this far, by seeking understanding, by holding onto hope even when answers were hard to find.

Some days, you might feel like you are going backward. Some nights, your symptoms may feel overwhelming. In those times, remember that healing does not move in a straight line. It is more like a spiral. You might revisit old challenges, but each time you do, you have more tools, more wisdom, and more strength.

Your story is still unfolding. And though MCAS may shape its contours, it does not define its core. At the heart of your story is not illness, but you: your courage, your creativity, your persistence, your capacity for love and for living a life that matters.

Keep moving forward, one step at a time. Listen to your body's signals. Rely on your support team. Stay flexible with your plan. And remember to pause and notice the beauty around you, like flowers growing in the cracks, a stranger's kindness, or small victories that are worth celebrating.

This is not the end of your journey. It is a new beginning, one where you are equipped not just with information, but with perspective, encouragement, and the tools to shape a life that feels steady, meaningful, and yours.

May you use this knowledge as a compass, guiding you as you patiently tend your own garden, knowing that each season brings something new. Always remember: you are more than this condition, and your life can hold beauty, purpose, and peace, right here and right now.

Reflection & Journaling Prompts

To help carry this book into your daily life, here are a few gentle prompts you can use for reflection. You might write them down, record them as voice notes, or simply sit with them in quiet thought:

1. **What brings me comfort right now?** List small practices, foods, spaces, or people that help you feel safe and cared for.
2. **Where do I feel most supported?** Reflect on who in your life understands your journey, and how you might lean on them more.
3. **What small step could I take this week to feel steadier?** Think of one manageable action—a food to try, a walk to take, a practice to return to.
4. **What do I want to remember on hard days?** Write yourself a note of encouragement, the kind you'd give a dear friend, and keep it where you can return to it when symptoms flare.
5. **What vision of life am I moving toward?** Picture not just a life without symptoms, but a life with meaning, joy, and connection. Describe what it looks and feels like.

"When you help someone up a hill, you get closer to the top yourself."
– Norman Schwarzkopf

Let's make living with MCAS a little easier—together.
If this book helped you understand your body, calm a flare, or feel more in control, please take a moment to leave a short review—it truly helps others find their way, too.

Help someone else find answers faster.
Remind another reader they're not alone.
Keep this book visible for those who need it most.

Thank you for being part of this growing circle of understanding and support—helping more people live steadier, better lives, one story at a time.

With gratitude,
Kathleen Dodwell

Follow the link or scan the code to leave your review -
https://mybook.to/jBGj

Glossary

- **Antihistamines** – Medications that block the action of histamine, helping to reduce symptoms like itching, flushing and nasal congestion.
- **Bucket Effect** – Your body has a limited capacity for stressors—like a bucket that can only hold so much.
- **Corticosteroids** – Anti-inflammatory medications that suppress the immune system and can reduce mast cell activity; used for severe flares.
- **Cromolyn** – A mast cell stabilizer medication that reduces mast cell degranulation and is taken orally or inhaled.
- **Cytokines** – Small proteins released by immune cells that facilitate communication and drive inflammation.
- **DAO (diamine oxidase)** – An enzyme produced in the gut that breaks down ingested histamine; supplementation may help with histamine intolerance.
- **Degranulation** – The process by which mast cells release their chemical mediators into surrounding tissue.
- **Ehlers–Danlos syndrome (EDS)** – A group of genetic disorders affecting connective tissue, sometimes associated with MCAS.
- **Epinephrine (adrenaline)** – A hormone and emergency medication used to treat severe allergic reactions and anaphylaxis by relaxing airway muscles and tightening blood vessels.
- **H1 antihistamines** – Drugs that block histamine at H1 receptors to relieve symptoms like itching, sneezing and runny nose (e.g., cetirizine,

loratadine).

- **H2 antihistamines** – Drugs that block histamine at H2 receptors to reduce stomach acid and help with heartburn or gastric symptoms (e.g., ranitidine, famotidine).
- **Histamine** – A chemical released by mast cells that triggers inflammation and allergy symptoms such as itching, flushing and swelling.
- **Immunoglobulins (IgE, IgG, IgA)** – Types of antibodies produced by the immune system; IgE is involved in allergic reactions.
- **Ketotifen** – Another mast cell stabilizer that also acts as an antihistamine; often used for allergic conditions.
- **Leukotriene inhibitors** – Medications that block leukotrienes, inflammatory chemicals released by immune cells; often used for asthma (e.g., montelukast).
- **MCAS (Mast Cell Activation Syndrome)** – A condition in which mast cells are easily triggered to release chemicals, leading to widespread symptoms.
- **Mast cell stabilizers** – Medications such as cromolyn sodium and ketotifen that help prevent mast cells from releasing their chemicals.
- **Mast cells** – Immune cells that release chemicals like histamine and play a key role in allergic and inflammatory reactions.
- **Mastocytosis** – A disease involving the accumulation of abnormal mast cells in the skin or other organs; distinct from MCAS.
- **Mediators** – Substances released by mast cells (such as histamine, prostaglandins, tryptase) that cause symptoms of MCAS.
- **NSAIDs (Nonsteroidal anti-inflammatory drugs)** – Medications like ibuprofen that reduce inflammation and pain but may trigger reactions in some people with MCAS.
- **POTS (Postural Orthostatic Tachycardia Syndrome)** – A condition characterized by a significant increase in heart rate upon standing, sometimes seen with MCAS.
- **Prostaglandins** – Lipid compounds that act like hormones and contribute to inflammation and pain.
- **Quercetin** – A plant-derived flavonoid supplement that may help stabilize

mast cells and reduce inflammation.

- **Tachycardia** – An abnormally rapid heart rate.
- **Tryptase** – An enzyme released by mast cells; elevated levels in blood can indicate mast cell activation.
- **Yellow lights** – Early warning signs.

References

Understanding MCAS - From Symptoms to Diagnosis

1.1 What is Mast Cell Activation Syndrome?

(1). "Mast Cell Activation Syndrome (MCAS)." 2025. https://www.healthline.com/health/mast-cell-activation-syndrome

(2). (n.d.). *Systemic mastocytosis - Symptoms and causes.* Mayo Clinic. https://www.mayoclinic.org/diseases-conditions/systemic-mastocytosis/symptoms-causes/syc-20352859

(3). "A simpler path to answers for patients with mast cell activation syndrome." Mayo Clinic Laboratories. 2025. https://news.mayocliniclabs.com/2025/08/11/a-simpler-path-to-answers-for-patients-with-mast-cell-activation-syndrome/

(4). "Mastocytosis and Mast Cell Activation Disorders: Clearing the Air." *International Journal of Molecular Sciences* 22 (2020). https://www.mdpi.com/1422-0067/22/20/11270

1.2 Recognizing the Signs and Symptoms

(1). "Postural orthostatic tachycardia syndrome (POTS): State of the science and clinical care from a 2019 National Institutes of Health Expert Consensus Meeting - Part 1." *Autonomic Neuroscience: Basic and Clinical* 235 (2021): 102868. https://pubmed.ncbi.nlm.nih.gov/33980338/

(2). Weinstock, Leonard B., Nelson, Renee M., Blitshteyn, and Svetlana. "Neuropsychiatric Manifestations of Mast Cell Activation Syndrome and

Response to Mast-Cell-Directed Treatment: A Case Series." *Journal of Personalized Medicine* 13 (2023). https://doi.org/10.3390/jpm13111562

(3). "POTS and MCAS: What is the link?." 2023. https://www.eds.clinic/articles/mast-cell-activation-syndrome-postural-orthostatic-tachycardia-syndrome

(4). Kotha, Archana; Bruno, Katelyn; Fairweather, and DeLisa. "Mast cell disorders in Ehlers-Danlos syndrome." *American Journal of Medical Genetics: Seminars in Medical Genetics* 174 (2017). https://pubmed.ncbi.nlm.nih.gov/28261938/

(5). "New Allergies or Food Intolerance After COVID-19? Mast Cell and Histamine Issues." 2024. https://longcovidjustice.org/mcas/

1.3 Diagnosis and Medical Testing

(1). "Testing | Mast Cell Action." https://www.mastcellaction.org/testing

(2). "Tryptase levels as an indicator of mast-cell activation in systemic anaphylaxis and mastocytosis." *Journal of Clinical Investigation* 82 (1988). https://pubmed.ncbi.nlm.nih.gov/3295549/

(3). "Mastocytosis and Mast Cell Activation Disorders: Clearing the Air." *Journal of Allergy and Clinical Immunology* 144. https://pmc.ncbi.nlm.nih.gov/articles/PMC8540348/

(4). "Mast Cell Activation Syndrome (MCAS): Symptoms & Treatment." Cleveland Clinic. 2023. https://my.clevelandclinic.org/health/diseases/mast-cell-activation-syndrome

(5). "The Provider Primer Series: Mediator testing - Mast Attack." 2016. https://www.mastattack.org/2016/10/the-provider-primer-series-mediator-testing/

(6). Klimas, and Lisa. "Chromogranin A." 2017. https://www.mastattack.org/2017/02/chromogranin-a/

Conventional Medical Treatments

2.1 Medications Commonly Used

(1). Baroody, M., F., Naclerio & M., R. (2000). *Antiallergic effects of H1-receptor antagonists.* Allergy 55. https://pubmed.ncbi.nlm.nih.gov/11291777/

(2). (2023). *H2 Blockers - StatPearls.* https://www.ncbi.nlm.nih.gov/books/NBK525994/

(3). (1982). *Antiallergic drug cromolyn may inhibit histamine secretion by regulating phosphorylation of a mast cell protein.* Journal of Immunology 128. https://pubmed.ncbi.nlm.nih.gov/6153130/

(4). (n.d.). *Ketotifen | Advanced Drug Monograph.* MedPath. https://trial.medpath.com/drug/report/77f2fb1f8533c87a

(5). (2025). *The Provider Primer Series: Mediator testing.* mastattack.org. https://www.mastattack.org/2016/10/the-provider-primer-series-mediator-testing/

(6). (2025). *Mast Cell Activation Syndrome (MCAS): Symptoms & Treatment.* Cleveland Clinic. https://my.clevelandclinic.org/health/diseases/mast-cell-activation-syndrome

(7). (n.d.). *What is Mast Cell Activation Syndrome (MCAS)?.* allergyasthmanetwork.org. https://allergyasthmanetwork.org/mast-cell-diseases/mcas/

2.2 Other Medical & Emerging Approaches

(1). (2023). *Thymosin α1 and Its Role in Viral Infectious Diseases: The Mechanism and Clinical Application.* https://pubmed.ncbi.nlm.nih.gov/37110771/

(2). (n.d.). *Vasoactive intestinal peptide.* https://en.wikipedia.org/wiki/Vasoactive_intestinal_peptide

(3). (2025). *KPV: The Future of Anti-Inflammatory Research.* https://www.labofrad.com/peptideinfo/kpv/

(4). (n.d.). *FAQ About Biologic Medication.* https://biologicmeds.org/faqs-about-biologics/

(5). (n.d.). *IVIG | RDS.* https://www.rheumaderm-society.org/ivig/

(6). (n.d.). *Mast Cell Activation Syndrome (MCAS) - Everything You Need to Know*. https://integrative-medicine.ca/mast-cell-activation-syndrome-everything-you-need-to-know/

2.4 Working with Healthcare Providers

(1). Highsmith & M., J. (2019). *Steroid-induced Secondary Osteoporosis*. https://www.healthcentral.com/condition/spinal-fractures/steroid-induced-secondary-osteoporosis

Natural Therapies and Lifestyle Strategies

3.1 Dietary Approaches

(1). (n.d.). *Why Are Leftovers High In Histamine?*. https://wellwisp.com/why-are-leftovers-high-in-histamine/

(2). (n.d.). *Supplements for MCAS and Histamine Intolerance*. https://www.eds.clinic/articles/supplements-for-mcas-and-histamine-intolerance

3.2 Natural and Complementary Therapies

(1). Zhao, Y. & al., e. (2024). *Quercetin Attenuates MRGPRX2-Mediated Mast Cell Degranulation via the MyD88/IKK/NF-κB and PI3K/AKT/Rac1/Cdc42 Pathway*. Frontiers in Pharmacology 15. https://pubmed.ncbi.nlm.nih.gov/39398230/

(2). (2015). *Frequent ingestion of the curry spice curcumin inhibits mast cell expansion and suppresses intestinal anaphylaxis in a murine model of food allergy*. Journal of Immunology 190. https://academic.oup.com/jimmunol/article/190/Supplement_1/59.18/8000145

(3). (2025). *Stabilizing effect of green tea extract and epigallocatechin-3-gallate (EGCG) on mast cell: an in vivo study*. https://pubmed.ncbi.nlm.nih.gov/40533674/

(4). Majeed, M., Nagabhushanam, R., Lawrence, R., Nallathambi, R., Thiyagarajan, S., Mundkur & L. (2021). *Boswellia serrata Extract Containing 30% 3-Acetyl-11-Keto-Boswellic Acid Attenuates Inflammatory Mediators and Preserves Extracellular Matrix in Collagen-Induced Arthritis*. Journal of

Ethnopharmacology 276. https://pubmed.ncbi.nlm.nih.gov/34650445/

(5). (n.d.). *Supplements and MCAS.* https://www.mastcellaction.org/supplements-and-mcas

(6). Schnedl, J., W., Enko & Dietmar. (2021). *Histamine Intolerance Originates in the Gut.* Intestinal Disorders 5. https://pubmed.ncbi.nlm.nih.gov/33921522/

(7). (n.d.). *Mindfulness and Mental Health.* https://www.mastcellaction.org/mindfulness-and-mental-health

3.3 Environmental and Lifestyle Modifications

(1). (2025). *Managing your environment.* Mast Cell Action. https://www.mastcellaction.org/managing-your-environment

(2). (n.d.). *Managing your environment.* https://www.mastcellaction.org/managing-your-environment

(3). Johansson & Olle. (2000). *Electromagnetic fields and mast cells: a theoretical model to explain the sensitivity to electric and/or magnetic fields in humans.* Electromagnetic fields and mast cells: a theoretical model to explain the sensitivity to electric and/or magnetic fields in humans. Medical Hypotheses 55. https://pubmed.ncbi.nlm.nih.gov/10859662/

(4). Harvima, T, I., Nilsson & Gunnar. (2012). *Stress, the neuroendocrine system and mast cells: current understanding of their role in psoriasis.* Expert Review of Clinical Immunology 8. https://www.ovid.com/journals/excim/fulltext/10.1586/eci.12.1~stress-the-neuroendocrine-system-and-mast-cells-current

(5). (n.d.). *Nature and Mental Health.* Minnesota Department of Health. https://www.health.state.mn.us/communities/mentalhealth/nature.html

Medical Disclaimer

The content in this book is provided for general educational purposes only. It does not establish a doctor–patient relationship and should not be used as a substitute for personalized medical advice, diagnosis, or treatment. Always consult a qualified healthcare professional before starting, stopping, or changing any medication, supplement, diet, or therapy.

Discussions of medications, supplements, and procedures—including off-label or emerging uses—reflect the author's understanding at the time of publication. Evidence evolves, and recommendations may change. Drug names, dosages, contraindications, and interactions may vary by individual and by country; consult your clinician and local guidelines.

If you have a medical emergency (for example, signs of anaphylaxis such as trouble breathing, swelling of the lips or tongue, or severe dizziness), call your local emergency number immediately.

The author and publisher disclaim any liability for outcomes resulting from the use of information contained in this book.

www.ingramcontent.com/pod-product-compliance
Lightning Source LLC
LaVergne TN
LVHW090410210926
848480LV00002B/519